MW01273354

Okanagan Mission Secondary
4544 Gordon Drive
Kelowna, B.C. V1W 1T4

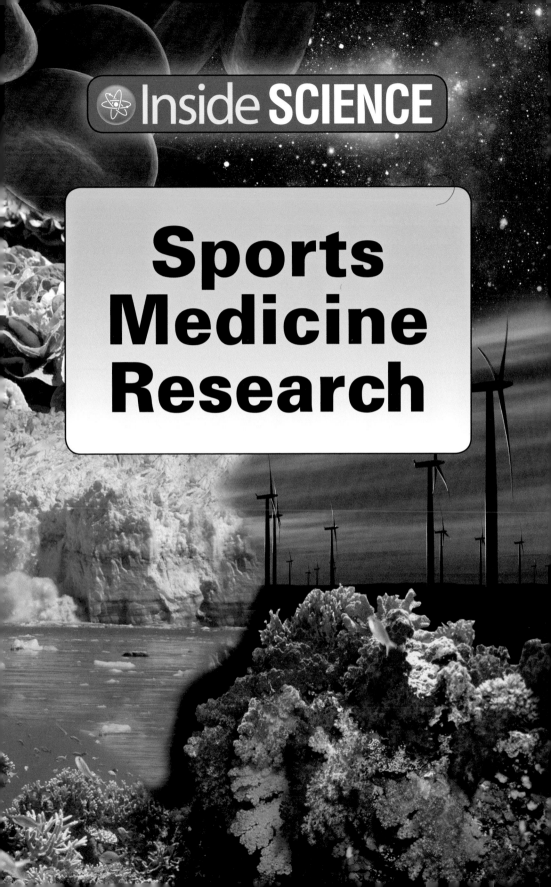

Inside SCIENCE

Sports Medicine Research

Other titles in the *Inside Science* series:

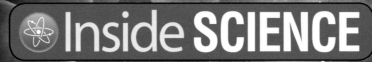

Sports
Medicine
Research

Gail B. Stewart

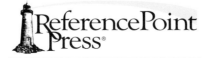

San Diego, CA

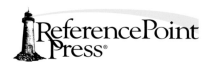

© 2013 ReferencePoint Press, Inc.
Printed in the United States

For more information, contact:
ReferencePoint Press, Inc.
PO Box 27779
San Diego, CA 92198
www.ReferencePointPress.com

LIBRARY OF CONGRESS CATALOGING-IN-PUBLICATION DATA

Stewart, Gail B. (Gail Barbara), 1949-
  Sports medicine research / Gail B. Stewart.
    p. cm. -- (Inside science series)
  Includes bibliographical references and index.
  ISBN-13: 978-1-60152-464-5 (hardback)
  ISBN-10: 1-60152-464-1 (hardback)
  1. Sports medicine--Research. I. Title.
  RC1210.S786 2012
  617.1'027072--dc23

                                                                    2012011480

Contents

Foreword

I n 2008, when the Yale Project on Climate Change and the George Mason University Center for Climate Change Communication asked Americans, "Do you think that global warming is happening?" 71 percent of those polled—a significant majority—answered "yes." When the poll was repeated in 2010, only 57 percent of respondents said they believed that global warming was happening. Other recent polls have reported a similar shift in public opinion about climate change.

Although respected scientists and scientific organizations worldwide warn that a buildup of greenhouse gases, mainly caused by human activities, is bringing about potentially dangerous and long-term changes in Earth's climate, it appears that doubt is growing among the general public. What happened to bring about this change in attitude over such a short period of time? Climate change skeptics claim that scientists have greatly overstated the degree and the dangers of global warming. Others argue that powerful special interests are minimizing the problem for political gain. Unlike experiments conducted under strictly controlled conditions in a lab or petri dish, scientific theories, facts, and findings on such a critical topic as climate change are often subject to personal, political, and media bias—whether for good or for ill.

At its core, however, scientific research is not about politics or 30-second sound bites. Scientific research is about questions and measurable observations. Science is the process of discovery and the means for developing a better understanding of ourselves and the world around us. Science strives for facts and conclusions unencumbered by bias, distortion, and political sensibilities. Although sometimes the methods and motivations are flawed, science attempts to develop a body of knowledge that can guide decision makers, enhance daily life, and lay a foundation to aid future generations.

The relevance and the implications of scientific research are profound, as members of the National Academy of Sciences point out in the 2009 edition of *On Being a Scientist: A Guide to Responsible Conduct in Research:*

Some scientific results directly affect the health and well-being of individuals, as in the case of clinical trials or toxicological studies. Science also is used by policy makers and voters to make informed decisions on such pressing issues as climate change, stem cell research, and the mitigation of natural hazards. . . . And even when scientific results have no immediate applications—as when research reveals new information about the universe or the fundamental constituents of matter—new knowledge speaks to our sense of wonder and paves the way for future advances.

The *Inside Science* series provides students with a sense of the painstaking work that goes into scientific research—whether its focus is microscopic cells cultured in a lab or planets far beyond the solar system. Each book in the series examines how scientists work and where that work leads them. Sometimes, the results are positive. Such was the case for Edwin McClure, a once-active high school senior diagnosed with multiple sclerosis, a degenerative disease that leads to difficulties with coordination, speech, and mobility. Thanks to stem cell therapy, in 2009 a healthier McClure strode across a stage to accept his diploma from Virginia Commonwealth University. In some cases, cutting-edge experimental treatments fail with tragic results. This is what occurred in 1999 when 18-year-old Jesse Gelsinger, born with a rare liver disease, died four days after undergoing a newly developed gene therapy technique. Such failures may temporarily halt research, as happened in the Gelsinger case, to allow for investigation and revision. In this and other instances, however, research resumes, often with renewed determination to find answers and solve problems.

Through clear and vivid narrative, carefully selected anecdotes, and direct quotations each book in the *Inside Science* series reinforces the role of scientific research in advancing knowledge and creating a better world. By developing an understanding of science, the responsibilities of the scientist, and how scientific research affects society, today's students will be better prepared for the critical challenges that await them. As members of the National Academy of Sciences state: "The values on which science is based—including honesty, fairness, collegiality, and openness—serve as guides to action in everyday life as well as in research. These values have helped produce a scientific enterprise of unparalleled usefulness, productivity, and creativity. So long as these values are honored, science—and the society it serves—will prosper."

Important Events in Sports Medicine Research

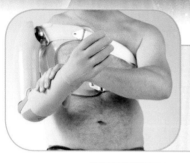

1955
The first myoelectric prosthetic arm is introduced, enabling the wearer to control the prosthetic by means of electrodes placed inside the sleeve, over the muscles of the stump.

1965
A British sports council funds a study of the effects of altitude on runners, in preparation for the 1968 summer Olympics in Mexico City.

1924
Alexander Maximow discovers a type of adult stem cell that can be helpful in healing damaged tissue.

1900	1930	1960	1990

1865
The end of the American Civil War, a war that resulted in lost limbs for 60,000 to 70,000 soldiers, spurs a number of advances in prostheses that will one day also benefit many athletes.

1928
The International Olympic Committee officially establishes the International Federation of Sports Medicine (FIMS) to engage physicians in healing and helping to prevent sports injuries and in sharing research.

1984
Van Phillips, an amputee, begins selling his innovative Flex-Foot prostheses that allow athletes missing a leg to compete with nonamputees.

1974
Orthopedic surgeon Frank Jobe performs the first UCL (ulnar collateral ligament) reconstruction surgery, known afterward as "Tommy John surgery," enabling pitcher Tommy John to continue another 14 years in baseball.

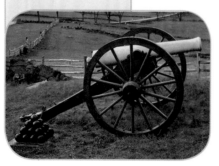

IMPORTANT EVENTS

1993
The ImPACT test, developed by neuropsychologist Mark Lovell and neurosurgeon Joseph Maroon, is used for the first time to determine whether an athlete can return to sports after a concussion.

2007
Todd Kuiken pioneers a revolutionary surgical technique called targeted muscle reinnervation (TMR) that will eventually enable amputees to control a prosthetic arm with their thoughts.

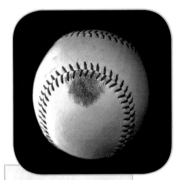

2000
The Fox Point–Bayside School District outside Milwaukee votes to require middle school soccer players to wear leather helmets to protect them from concussions.

2005
Massachusetts voters reject a law making it mandatory for school soccer players to wear helmets.

2010
Yankees pitcher Bartolo Colón receives a stem cell injection to heal connective tissue in his pitching arm.

1995   1999   2003   2007   2011

1999
Platelet-rich plasma therapy is used for the first time by oral surgeons and plastic surgeons to stimulate healing.

2011
An autopsy of the brain of 28-year-old NHL player Derek Boogaard determines that he is the youngest player known to have suffered from chronic traumatic encephalopathy.

2012
The Mayo Clinic releases the results of a study showing that platelet-rich plasma therapy helps to break up scar tissue in a human tendon.

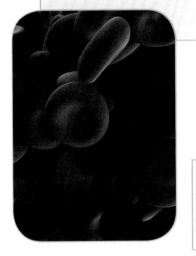

2002
An autopsy of former NFL player Mike Webster finds evidence of chronic traumatic encephalopathy, a degenerative brain disease found in athletes and others who suffer repetitive brain injury. This marks the first time an athlete other than a boxer is found to have the disease.

Getting Back in the Game

On December 30, 2011, Jack Jablonski, a Minnesota high school hockey forward from Benilde–St. Margaret's High School, was critically injured. As he raced toward a puck near the opponents' goal, Jack was pursued by two opposing players. The first hit him between the shoulder blades, after which the second slammed him into the boards. The hits, which are illegal in high school hockey, ended with 16-year-old Jack lying face down, motionless, on the ice.

His father, Mike Jablonski, says it was a parent's worst nightmare. "Anybody . . . who's ever had a son who played hockey or football, when your son goes down in that type of situation, you say, 'OK, get up,'"[1] he says. But Jack did not get up. He did not even move. When it seemed apparent that something was seriously wrong, Jablonski rushed from the stands down to the ice and crouched down next to his son. "He just said, 'Dad, I can't feel anything,'"[2] says Jablonski."

> **prognosis**
>
> The prospect of recovery as anticipated from the usual course of an injury, disease, or other medical condition.

A Bleak Prognosis

Jack was rushed to the hospital, where doctors announced that they believed he had fractured two vertebrae and had severed his spinal cord. The prognosis seemed even bleaker a week later, after the surgery that fused the two vertebrae. Doctors explained to the family that surgery could not fix the type of spinal injury Jack suffered and that the 16-year-old athlete might never walk again.

After performing the fusing procedure, neurosurgeon Walter Galicich explained to the media that the extent of the spinal cord damage made him less than hopeful about Jack's recovery. "God willing, there will be some improvement over the next few weeks, but at this point we really haven't seen any significant improvement and unfortunately we don't expect him to get much function back. Hopefully (Jack) proves me wrong. I would like nothing better."[3]

Jack's family remained hopeful, saying that Jack was a fighter. "This news is devastating to Jack and everyone who loves him," they announced on the family's website. "Our hope and dream is that he will be able to prove this prognosis wrong. Our priority is to help Jack accept and transition into his new life, a life that we did not plan, but one that we have to embrace."[4]

Millions of Injuries

The Centers for Disease Control and Prevention (CDC) estimates that 7.1 million Americans suffer sports- or exercise-related injuries each year. Most are not as life-changing as the one suffered by Jack Jablonski. However, they can still be painful and debilitating enough to prevent athletes from participating in the sport they love or get paid to play. Sports news

Visiting hockey players stop by the hospital to see Jack Jablonski, who was paralyzed as a result of spinal cord damage sustained during a high school ice hockey game. Sports medicine researchers in various fields are working to improve prevention and treatment of all sorts of sports injuries.

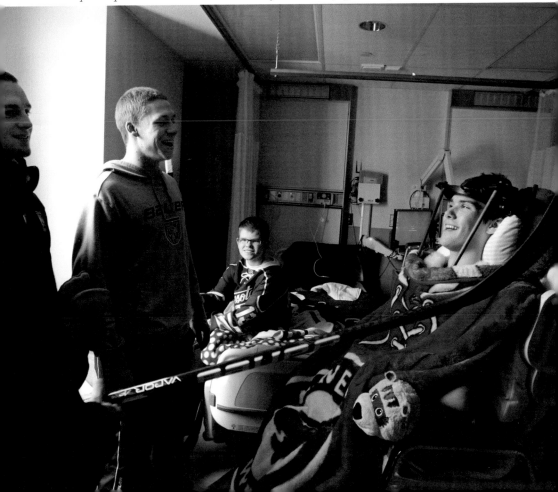

reports are filled with evidence of this: professional football players sidelined with concussions or torn knee ligaments, baseball pitchers sitting out a season recuperating from elbow or shoulder trouble, and golfers plagued by back injuries.

And it is not only adults and professional athletes who endure painful sports injuries. In the United States, approximately 40 million children and teenagers participate in some type of organized athletics. In 2009 nearly 3.7 million of them were seen in hospital emergency rooms for sports-related injuries. And, according to the CDC data, those numbers do not include those whose injuries did not result in an emergency room visit or who saw their family doctor instead.

> ## ligament
>
> A band of tough, fibrous connective tissue that connects two bones or holds a joint together.

Benefiting People

Researchers throughout the world are working to find ways to treat and prevent sports injuries of all kinds. Ann McKee, a concussion and brain injury researcher at Boston University School of Medicine, is one of these researchers. She led a 2010 study that examined the brains of athletes who suffered numerous head injuries playing hockey or football. The findings of the study provided important information about the nature of the damage sustained in traumatic brain injury cases—whether they occur on the battlefield in Afghanistan or playing football. "Future work based on these observations offers a significant opportunity to develop treatments to benefit veterans and all Americans well into the future," she said, adding, "We can't treat what we don't understand."[5]

Sometimes the athletes themselves drive research in sports medicine. A rapidly growing segment of the population is adults between 45 and 65, often referred to as "baby boomers." According to sports physician Ted Parks, chief of staff at Denver's Colorado Orthopedic and Surgical Hospital, they are athletic in ways former generations had never been at that age. "We're seeing sports injuries in people in their late 40s and 50s that we used to see only in high school, college, or professional athletes," he says. "[They] are out there playing and competing, and when they get hurt, they want to get fixed and back to the game ASAP."[6]

That has resulted in a quickly growing number of patients needing the services of sports physicians and has brought a whole new set of challenges for those doctors. According to Andy Pruitt of the Boulder Center for Sports Medicine, "The baby boomers and their beat-up skeletons have driven a whole new industry. There are new medical journals and organizations, injectable lubricants for knees, high-tech braces, and new minimally invasive surgical techniques all aimed at them."[7]

But no matter what motivates researchers, every day millions of athletes benefit from the innovation of doctors, engineers, chemists, surgeons, and physical therapists. The work they do has given athletes new ways to stay healthy, to train in smarter and more productive ways, and even to recover from injuries that once meant the curtailment of athletic life.

What Is Sports Medicine?

Sam Alder knew something was wrong just as he was beginning his six-mile run (9.7 km) through his west Chicago suburban neighborhood. "I'd just started off, and all of a sudden I felt a really sharp pain in my calf," the 21-year-old says. "Right away I felt that my whole lower leg was incredibly stiff. I've been running since junior high school, but I've never felt anything like that before—it was like a stabbing pain. It was clear after a few minutes that no amount of warming up was going to help my leg loosen up. Actually, what seemed strange to me was that walking and stretching seemed to make the pain worse."[8]

Alder went home and tried icing his leg, and when that did not help, he tried heat. Realizing that the pain was not subsiding, he made an appointment that afternoon with his doctor, a specialist in sports medicine. "Right away she said she suspected it was a calf sprain, just by the symptoms and the location of the pain," says Alder. "She did an MRI [magnetic resonance imaging scan] and that showed that I had several small tears in the muscle. She told me that it would be probably between 4 to 6 weeks before I could even think about starting to run again."[9]

Though the injury was not catastrophic, Alder admits he was extremely frustrated and disappointed by the diagnosis because he had been training for his first marathon.

> I'd been working very hard to get in shape to run the Chicago Marathon in October. I knew taking a month or more off with this calf sprain was going to completely derail the marathon thing, at least for this year, and so the news was really hard to take. At least I knew what it was, though, and it was something I would hopefully bounce back from if I took care of it. My goal now is next year's marathon. I'm kind of depressed that I won't be running this year, but I'm grateful I have a doctor who knows what she's doing.[10]

An Ancient Branch of Medicine

Sports medicine is the branch of medicine that aims to maintain the health of athletes as well as to diagnose and treat the injuries and conditions that can occur in people who participate in athletics. Though sports medicine did not emerge as a specialty in medical schools around the world until the 1970s, sports medicine actually has very old beginnings.

Herodicus, a Greek physician who lived in the fifth century BC, is widely considered "the father of modern sports medicine." It was Herodicus who first suggested combining athletics with scientific knowledge in order to get the best results in sporting contests. Serving as a trainer and physician for wrestlers, boxers, and runners, he urged the athletes in his care to warm up before matches so that their muscles would be limber and less likely to become torn or sprained. He was the first to advocate the application of heat to aching muscles. He urged athletes who were ill to sit in steam rooms to help them recover more quickly. The Greek philosopher Plato wrote that it was not until Herodicus that "doctors made use of the modern methods of nursing disease."[11]

magnetic resonance imaging

A scan using a magnetic field to take pictures of soft tissue, such as organs and muscles.

The ancient Romans loved watching sports, too, albeit more violent sports, such as gladiators fighting one another, chariot races, and wrestling matches between men and wild animals. Galen, a noted Greek physician working in Rome during the second century AD, worked as both a trainer and physician at a large gladiator school in Asia Minor. Galen's interest in athletics extended beyond training; he also took an interest in the recommended diet of the gladiators.

According to historian Michael Grant, "Gladiators were called *hordearii*, barley men, because of the amount of barley that they ate, a muscle-building food."[12] Galen disagreed with a diet heavy on barley, however. He felt such a diet made the men's flesh soft.

Sports Medicine

After the fall of the Roman Empire in AD 476, organized athletics all but disappeared. In fact, it was not until the late nineteenth century—more than 1,400 years later—that sporting events became widespread in Europe and the United States. Most of these events were games between teams representing colleges and universities. As the competition increased, so did the injuries. More and more teams began hiring trainers who had some background in first aid.

Sports medicine was officially recognized as a science by the modern Olympic Games in 1928, when a committee was formed to organize

High school basketball players demonstrate their talents on the court. Millions of adults and young people now take part in school and recreational sports. While this participation is good for overall health and fitness it has also resulted in a rise in sports injuries.

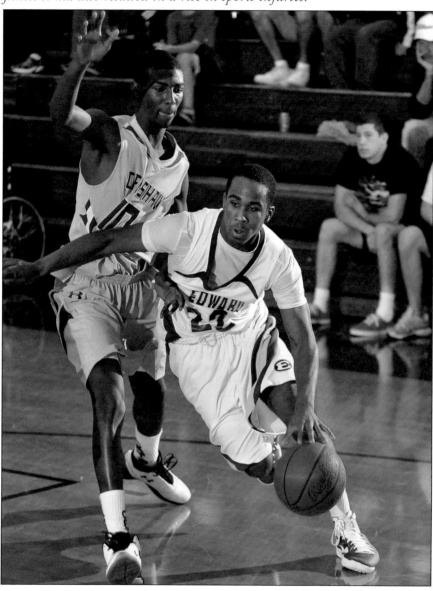

what came to be called the International Federation of Sports Medicine (FIMS), a group of experts in sports medicine from nations around the world. Physicians would take a role in healing injuries as well as preventing them. They would also strive to study sports injuries and work to find ways to prevent them. By the mid-1970s, many medical schools began offering sports medicine as a specialty field. Sports medicine in the twenty-first century involves a wide range of medical professionals, including sports medicine physicians, who specialize in fitness and injury prevention; orthopedists, who specialize in bones and joints; neurologists, who specialize in brain injuries; physical therapists; occupational therapists; chiropractors; athletic trainers; and others.

Increasing Numbers of Patients

But the biggest change over the centuries is the number of people who utilize the talents of professionals who deal with sports injuries. Much has changed since the days when sports were the domain of professional teams of elite athletes. Today, people of all ages and abilities participate in sports and exercise. In the United States, as many as 60 million adults say they exercise or play sports at least once a week, and 41 million children play at least one organized youth sport.

One big reason for the explosive growth in athletics, says Canadian athletic trainer Greg Pfiefer, is that people understand that exercising makes people healthier. "People get the message a sedentary lifestyle is not healthy, and that exercise and fitness are linked," he says. "And, just as important, they also have learned that you do not have to be really great at a sport to enjoy it. A lot of people have decided that it's more fun to play than to watch [games] on TV. So those who are just starting out in a tennis league, or taking up racquetball or walking on a regular basis, they can get the benefits of exercising, while having fun."[13]

But whether weekend joggers, Little Leaguers, or runners aspiring to compete in their first marathon, these people sometimes need medical care, just as the multimillion-dollar professional athletes do. With increasing frequency, sports medicine professionals are the ones they seek out, whether the issue is a twisted ankle, an aching elbow or knee, or something more serious. These specialists are the ones most likely to diagnose and treat their problems and get them back to their sports.

Should EMTs Remove Helmets?

Sometimes sports medicine research aims to assess particular techniques used by doctors, trainers, or others who help injured athletes. In a 2000 study at the University of Minnesota, scientists addressed the question of whether emergency medical technicians (EMTs) called to help a hockey player with a possible spinal cord injury should remove the player's helmet or leave it on as they transport the player to the hospital.

In the study, 10 adult men between 18 and 28 years old, without a spinal injury, were fitted with hockey pads and helmets. Afterward, each was strapped to a board used in cases of spinal cord injury to keep the head still. Wearing pads and helmet, then pads only, they were scanned with a sophisticated X-ray machine. The scans showed conclusively that considerable extension of the spine occurred when the player's helmet was removed. The findings of the study recommend that the helmet be kept on as the player is transported to the hospital because it keeps the head in a safer, neutral position. As a result of this study, EMTs are now trained not to remove an injured player's helmet in such situations.

Muscle Tears and Strains

The vast majority of the injuries sports medicine professionals see involve damage or stress to one of the 640 muscles that support the skeletal system. Sore knees, aching triceps, ankle sprains, and painful shoulder muscles are common complaints among athletes. Most of these can be treated with heat, ice, over-the-counter anti-inflammatory medications, and rest. Occasionally, however, the problem is more serious and requires medical help.

St. Paul police officer Brady Harrison, a former all-star member of the Indiana University wrestling team, recalls the moment he tore his right bicep, a muscle between the shoulder and the elbow:

> I was what we called "shooting a single leg," which means I put my head down and was aiming to grab my opponent's leg and take him down that way. I basically grabbed him with my right arm around his leg, and had my left arm locked with my right, for support. Anyway, my hand got stuck—my bicep stretched,

and I was bearing the guy's whole weight on my right shoulder. I could feel right away a slight sense that my shoulder was being stretched, almost dislocated. And then when I released the guy and stood up, I could feel the pain—a really severe burning that ran down my arm to my fingers. I was pretty sure something had ripped. It's been years, but I can still remember that it felt like someone had driven a Mack truck over my shoulder.[14]

Harrison says that his trainer ordered him to have an MRI done. An MRI, or magnetic resonance imaging, is a test that uses a magnetic field and pulses of radio wave energy to make pictures of organs and other structures inside the body. Unlike an X-ray, an MRI can clearly show damage to soft tissues such as the biceps tendons.

In Harrison's case, his doctor could see that the muscle was damaged and recommended arthroscopic surgery to fix it. "Basically what they do is make two small incisions—one on the front and one on the back parts of the shoulder," Harrison explains. "They put two tubes in, with little cameras, and they could see the bicep. They repaired it right then, and other than having to have my arm in a sling for six months, the procedure was pretty easy."[15]

> **arthroscopic surgery**
>
> A procedure in which a fiber-optic instrument is inserted through an incision near a joint and used to visually examine and repair damaged tissue.

Treating Disc Injuries

Some of the most painful injuries suffered by athletes involve the muscles or nerves around the spine. In some cases in which rest or medication cannot heal the injury, surgery is an option. In 2011 Martell Webster, a basketball player for the Minnesota Timberwolves, was experiencing pain in his lower back, which made it difficult to play. His doctors suspected that he might have a problem with a disc—a common injury among athletes.

The human spinal column is formed by small bones, or vertebrae, that are stacked on top of one another. Between each of the vertebrae is a thin disc made of cartilage that is filled with a jellylike center. The discs act much like shock absorbers, protecting the vertebrae from rubbing together. If one of these discs breaks, the spongy center can slip out of the disc, or herniate, and put pressure on the nerve roots of the spinal cord, causing a tremendous amount of discomfort. Tests showed that Webster did indeed have a herniated disk, which necessitated surgery.

More and more sports physicians are called on to do a surgical procedure called a microdiscectomy to help ease the pain of herniated discs. The surgeon makes a very small incision. That drastically reduces the chances of infection, since the wound is far smaller than in surgical wounds from traditional open surgery. A smaller incision also means that the athlete will have far less pain afterward and will almost always heal more quickly.

Using either a microscope or special goggles, the surgeon can work with precision, removing the parts of the soft center of the disc that are putting pressure on the nerve root. "We just take that fragment out," explains Dallas orthopedic surgeon Robert H. Henderson. "We make sure there aren't any other loose fragments, we also make sure that in the area there is no other impingement (impact) on the nerve root, which we can resect [trim away] with instruments. The pressure is off immediately."[16]

An Unlikely Sports Danger

When people think of sports injuries, a bacterial infection would rarely come to mind. However, in recent years bacteria called methicillin-resistant *Staphylococcus aureus*, often referred to as MRSA, has surfaced in the sports world. For years, this particular staph bacterium typically affected people in hospitals, nursing homes, and dialysis centers. With increasing frequency, however, MRSA has been infecting healthy people, especially athletes, and has been causing them to become very ill—and in a few cases, has caused deaths.

In 2008 a 16-year-old Los Angeles high school wrestler named Noah Armendariz died after being infected with MRSA. Soon after coming home from a wrestling camp, he developed flu-like symptoms. His body ached, he had a fever, and then four days later he broke out with a rash. At first doctors suspected chicken pox or perhaps an allergic reaction to a medication he was taking for a dislocated shoulder. Most frighteningly, according to his mother, was that Noah even had difficulty walking. "He was shuffling around like an old man,"[17] she recalls.

After several trips to the hospital, doctors finally diagnosed his illness as a staph infection. They explained that MRSA is dangerous because it

MRSA

A strain of staph bacteria that is resistant to many antibiotics.

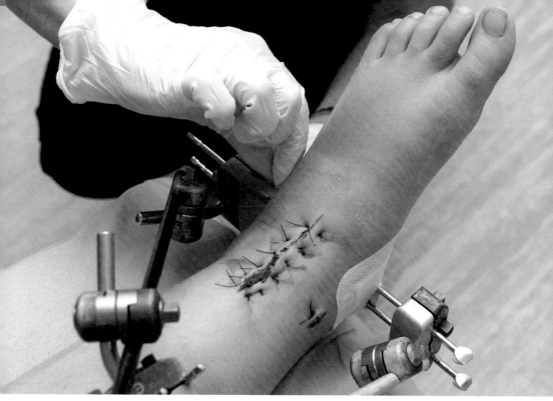

A patient who underwent surgery for a fractured ankle developed a MRSA infection. MRSA has claimed the lives of young athletes, and it presents serious challenges for medical researchers.

is resistant to many antibiotics and can quickly spread to the heart and lungs, where it can be fatal. In some cases an affected body part must be amputated so the bacteria cannot spread throughout the body. Tragically, the doctors were unable to save Noah when the staph spread to his heart.

The bacteria is commonly found on skin; to spread and enter the body it needs an open wound or abrasion on the skin. Artificial football turf, common in US high schools, can produce just the sort of abrasion that can harbor MRSA. More and more cases have been reported among football players and wrestlers, who often sustain wounds and experience a great deal of skin-to-skin contact. Doctors have found that MRSA can be spread in locker rooms, too, often by teammates sharing razors, towels, and even soap.

The Challenge of New Sports

In addition to being well versed on such diseases, surgery techniques, and a variety of procedures to help their patients, sports medicine professionals have had to stay abreast of new sports and the challenges those

Dangerous Cheerleading

A study completed in 2010 verified something sports medicine professionals already suspected—that cheerleading is one of the most dangerous sports for high school girls. The National Center for Catastrophic Sport Injury Research at the University of North Carolina found that cheerleaders suffer more than 65 percent of the dangerous injuries in girls' high school athletics—far more than hockey, basketball, and softball.

Frederick Mueller, director of the research center, says that he has tracked down 73 cases of catastrophic injuries in US cheerleaders since 1984. He defines catastrophic injuries as those causing permanent disabilities, such as fractured skulls and broken necks. Even two deaths occurred in that time period. The reason for those troubling statistics appears to be the changing nature of cheerleading—from girls singing and dancing with pom-poms to its current form, according to Mueller, "a gymnastics-type event where they're throwing girls 25–30 feet in the air—and sometimes missing them on the way down."

Researchers say that the stunts are usually done without safety mats, often on hard gym floors. And because cheerleading is not always categorized as an official sport, the safety measures required for other sports—trained coaches who act as spotters in practice and performances, for example—are often absent.

Quoted in Melissa Dahl, "Flying Without a Net: Cheer Injuries on the Rise," Fitness on msnbc.com, May 20, 2010. www.msnbc.msn.com.

sports present to athletes. For example, the first Ironman Triathlon held in Kona, Hawaii, in 1977 consisted of a 2.4-mile swim (3.8 km), a 112-mile bike ride (180.2 km), and a marathon run of 26.219 miles (42.1 km). No one could have predicted then the types of injuries or other medical issues that would surface in a sporting event held in the intense Hawaiian sun.

Each year the race grew more and more popular—from 15 entrants the first year in 1977 to 850 in 1982. But with hundreds of athletes suffering from dehydration, gastric distress, skin rashes, painful muscle spasms, and other complaints, the small contingent of doctors on duty were overwhelmed. Ironman officials realized they would need far more medical support for the athletes than Hawaii could provide.

To solve the problem, they decided to hold a medical symposium during the week of the race to lure sports physicians interested in research. "The race's rising reputation attracted top experts from around the world," writes Jené Shaw in *Inside Triathlon* magazine, "who were eager to see first-hand what the body went through when it endured 140.6 miles of exercise."[18]

Not only did the physicians who attended the symposium help out in the medical tent at the triathlon, but they also learned a great deal about the limits and problems faced by endurance athletes—problems that had never been researched. For example, they were the first to document something called exercise-related hyponatremia, a condition in which athletes under the extreme conditions of a triathlon sometimes take in too much water during exercise and unknowingly dilute the sodium in their bloodstreams. Sodium is vitally important to athletes; a sodium level that plummets can create problems with the athlete's blood pressure and nervous system.

hyponatremia

A metabolic condition in which there is not enough sodium, or salt, in the body fluids; it can result from drinking too much water during exercise and lead to mental confusion, convulsions, and muscle spasms.

Robert Laird, the first physician to assist in the Ironman Triathlons, says he is proud of the research that has come out of his experience with the event: "When we first started, there was just no information on endurance athletes. Now there's a huge wealth of it. . . . Most of your main researchers have been in the Kona medical tent here at least once. That's probably one of the things I'm proudest of—the dissemination of information on how to treat an athlete in distress."[19]

Research and Hope

But a range of other acute injuries or conditions has been a challenge to sports medicine researchers. A skier's severe knee injury, a soccer or football player's multiple concussions, the loss of a limb in a car accident, and other injuries can mean the end of an athlete's ability to play the sport he or she loves.

The future for these athletes depends on the work scientific researchers are doing. Every day, researchers are learning more about various sports and their impact on the human body, and they continue to find clues to hasten the healing of many. Successes often seem to come agonizingly slowly; nonetheless, they can and do occur. In fact, some of the most dramatic findings are perhaps the most improbable, as researchers are learning that it may soon be possible, even for those who never dreamed of being able to participate in athletics again, to not only play but perhaps even to win.

Concussion Research

One of the most talked-about topics in sports medicine is the prevalence of concussions. The study of concussions is relatively new; before the twenty-first century no one had any idea how common or insidious these injuries were.

"The coaches would say, 'Got your bell rung, didn't you?' or something like that," says Glenn Olsen, a Wisconsin farmer who played both football and baseball in college.

> That was back in the 80s. You got knocked in the head, you got up, feeling kind of woozy and unsteady, and your coach would tell you, 'Okay, sit down for a minute or two till you get those cobwebs out, and let me know when you can go back in.' It was just part of playing back then—no one thought much about it. As players, we didn't know any better, and evidently [the coaches] didn't either.[20]

A Rapid Brain Shift

Experts have a much better idea of what constitutes a concussion in 2012 than their predecessors did decades ago. According to one definition, a concussion is "any change in mental status, such as confusion, disorientation, headache, or dizziness following a hit or jolt."[21] Concussions may occur in automobile accidents, falls, and other traumatic events, but they are occurring more and more frequently in sports.

A concussion occurs when the head receives a jolt which causes the brain to move quickly and sometimes collide with the inside of the skull. When the brain shifts rapidly, the force of that shifting can break blood vessels and stretch or tear the delicate nerve cells that are vital to communication between the brain and the rest of the body. In some cases, the brain may swell—a condition that can lead to permanent brain damage or even death. Sometimes the signs of a concussion are so mild that no one notices anything unusual. Other times the symptoms are immediately obvious, as when an athlete struggles with a headache, impaired vision, difficulty speaking and understanding, and trouble balancing.

"That was me, nine years ago—the concussed girl who couldn't find her way to the sideline,"[22] says Eva Connor, now 26. Connor played soccer in suburban Denver for several years before suffering a serious concussion when she was 17:

> I went up for a header in a game, and collided with another player. It was ironic, because I'd always been a little gun shy about getting banged on the head, but in this case, I never hit my head at all. We bumped shoulders, I guess, and I fell backward. I didn't hit my head or anything—it was more like whiplash; that's what the coach later told me. I didn't get knocked out, but I felt so weird. I was dizzy and just kind of foggy, like I was in someone else's body. I walked off the field, but to the wrong side, where the other team was. [The opposing] coach walked me back over to my side of the field, because I didn't seem to understand what to do.[23]

Numbers Research

Some of the ongoing research on concussions deals with establishing an accurate number of their occurrences. According to a 2011 estimate by the CDC, between 1.8 million and 3.8 million sports-related concussions occur in the United States each year. One reason for the wide variance in these numbers, say experts, is that many concussions, such as Connor's, go unreported because many coaches, parents, and players mistakenly believe that concussions always bring on a loss of consciousness.

The most publicized concussions are those suffered by pro hockey and football players, but researchers stress that concussions can occur in any sport or recreational activity. While football, hockey, and soccer account for a large number of concussions, 34 percent of concussions occur in individual sports like skating and bicycling.

The CDC has determined that as many as 300,000 concussions occurred in young people under the age of 18 in 2005, and that number is growing. According to a 2010 study in the journal *Pediatrics*, the number of 8- to 13-year-olds visiting emergency rooms with concussions more than doubled between 1997 and 2005. That troubles neurologist Julian Baines of West Virginia University. "The immature brain is still develop-

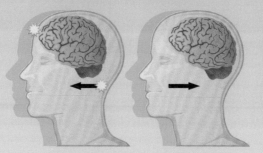

Concussions

As athletes get bigger, stronger, and faster than ever before, concussions—caused by violent collisions— have become a troubling part of many sports.

Concussions can occur when the brain moves inside the skull from an impact or whiplash effect.

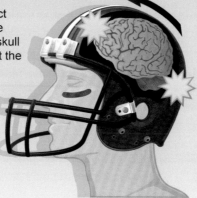

The force from the impact causes the brain to strike the inner surface of the skull and can rebound against the opposite side.

Symptoms
• Confusion
• Slurred speech
• Drowsiness
• Memory loss
• Blurred vision
• Bleeding nose or ears
• Seizures
• Nausea

Source: National Institutes of Health, "Concussion," 2012. www.nlm.nih.gov.

ing," he says. "That makes it more susceptible to damage and more likely to suffer repetitive injury."[24]

Post-Concussion Syndrome

Until the mid-1980s doctors believed that most concussions were temporary, that when the headache or blurry vision went away, any damage to the brain did, too. The prevailing wisdom among doctors was that when the symptoms disappeared, patients could return to their normal routine—including physical labor and sports—with no further problems.

However, research using rat models indicates that this is not the case. In several studies during the 1990s, rats were given concussions in a laboratory setting. Researchers noted that a concussion caused a sort of chemical burst within the rats' brains, which appeared to make the rats even more susceptible to getting another concussion. A second concussion, research showed, often had more a more serious outcome than the first. Sometimes it even resulted in death.

In 1993 a collision during a high school football game knocked Brandon Schultz of Anacortes, Washington, unconscious. Though he had severe headaches for the next week, he was back on the field for his school's next game. Ten minutes after making what onlookers said was a routine tackle, Schultz fell to the ground, convulsing in a seizure. He then went into a coma. Four emergency surgeries were necessary to reduce the pressure on his brain.

Schultz, today in his 30s, still has severe brain damage. He lives in his father's care and will likely never live alone. He has no peripheral vision, and his memory is poor. Schultz is not alone. Recent research shows that between 1997 and 2007, at least 50 American high school athletes died or were critically disabled from a head injury suffered in a football game.

second impact syndrome

A potentially life-threatening injury that can occur when an athlete sustains a concussion before symptoms from a previous concussion have completely disappeared.

Doctors now understand that though concussion symptoms may disappear, the structural damage to the brain caused by the concussion may not have disappeared. In that case, the athlete could possibly sustain a second, much more serious concussion from even a minor jolt. Second impact syndrome, or SIS, is rare, but the results are often death or permanent disability.

Ignoring Symptoms

For scientists, one of the most difficult aspects of concussion research is the realization that many cases of SIS could have been avoided. They have found that a lack of candor on the part of athletes about their head injuries results in many second concussions. Because an athlete who does not lose consciousness may not catch the eye of a coach or parent, it falls on the athlete to report it—something that many would not do.

"Young athletes are sometimes their own worst enemy," says St. Paul emergency medical technician (EMT) Ken Adams, who also teaches health professionals about concussions. "Most of them don't even know what a concussion is," he says.

Soccer and Concussions

As more research comes out showing the dangers of concussions, some experts worry about the repeated use of a player's head in soccer. A study in 2011 at the Albert Einstein College of Medicine at New York's Yeshiva University used a special MRI technique to do brain scans of 38 amateur soccer players, with an average age of 31. Afterward, the researchers conducted interviews with the players to find out how often in drills, practice, and games, they headed the ball.

After matching up the header frequencies to the brain scans, the scientists found more evidence of trauma in the scans of people who do the most headers. Further, they found that about 1,000 headers per year was the threshold after which they could view the damage. Further studies need to be done to assess the damage to younger players, whose brains are still developing.

"Repetitive heading could set off a cascade of responses that can lead to degeneration of brain cells," notes neuroscientist Michael Lipton, the author of the study. "Given that soccer is the most popular sport worldwide and is played extensively by children, these are findings that should be taken into consideration is order to protect soccer players."

Quoted in Ryan Jaslow, "Soccer Study Ties 'Heading' to Brain Damage," CBS News, November 29, 2011. www.cbsnews.com.

I read a recent study that suggests that only about 16 percent of college athletes know the symptoms of a concussion. A lot of them think you have to lose consciousness, but only 25 percent of concussions result in loss of consciousness. That means 75 percent of those concussions may not even be reported, because the athletes aren't aware they've had one.[25]

Adams says that young athletes may put their health at risk because they are too focused on their sport: "Think of it this way—if you're a high school kid and you get a concussion you may end up missing a season. So there goes your chance of maybe getting a scholarship. For a college kid, it's worse, because that kid might be looking at turning pro, and so he doesn't want to miss games. He'd rather keep playing than sit on the bench during a game, when scouts might be watching."[26]

Athletic Peer Pressure

Brian Howard, who played four years of football at Harvard, says that peer approval is just as critical for many athletes, and that the need to put up a strong front for one's teammates is very powerful. "Sure, there's pressure to not report concussions," he says. "You want a teammate who will line up every play, even when he's messed up. You know you can count on that guy. If you think that guy isn't going to play hard, or will pull himself out when he's hurt, down, or not 100 percent, then you don't want that guy lining up next to you."[27]

According to concussion expert Christopher Nowinski, some of that athletic peer pressure is institutionalized. "In many programs, injured athletes are forced to watch practice in full pads and helmets, while wearing a yellow or pink jersey over their regular practice jersey. . . . In reality, the jersey functions much like the 'Scarlet Letter.' The player might as well wear a flashing neon sign that says, 'I'm soft.'"[28]

chronic traumatic encephalopathy

A degenerative brain disease first noticed in boxers; it has been linked to depression, memory loss, and poor decision making.

One study led by neuropsychologist Michael McCrea interviewed 1,532 varsity football players from 20 high schools in the Milwaukee, Wisconsin, area. The study found that of those players suffering a concussion during the season, only 47.3 percent reported their injury. More than 41 percent admitted they did not report their concussions because they did not want to be withheld from competition.

Concussions and CTE

While most of the new concussion research is disturbing, none is more so than the research showing a link between athletes who sustain concussions and those suffering from a disease called chronic traumatic encephalopathy, or CTE. First noticed in the brains of boxers, the disease was commonly referred to as "punch-drunk syndrome." Those boxers who had been hit many times in their careers had some of the same symptoms as a heavy drinker would have—loss of balance, slow speech, and mental impairment. CTE is a degenerative disease that is linked to depression, memory loss, a tendency toward poor decision making, and Alzheimer's-like symptoms.

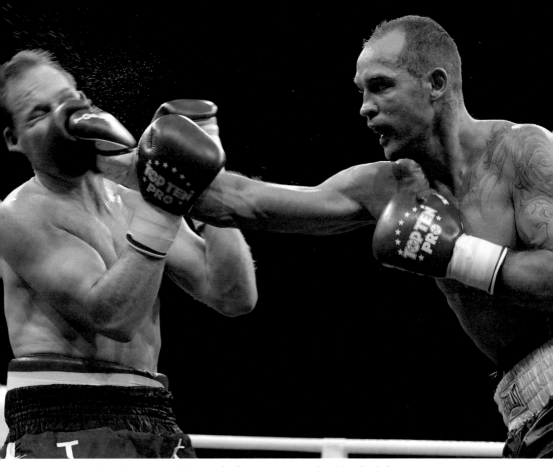

A boxer lands a painful punch during a match. The link between concussions in athletes and the degenerative disease known as CTE was first noticed in the brains of boxers. Constant battering of the head can lead to depression, memory loss, and Alzheimer's-like symptoms.

In 2002 a young Pittsburgh pathologist working for the coroner's office was assigned to perform the autopsy of 50-year-old Mike Webster, a retired NFL Hall of Fame player with the Pittsburgh Steelers. Pathologist Bennet Omalu had heard the news of Webster's death on the radio that morning and was struck by the sad life Webster had lived after football. According to the Associated Press: "Webster was diagnosed with brain damage in 1999, an injury caused by all the years of taking shots to the head. . . . The progressively worsening injury caused him to behave erratically, and Webster briefly was homeless, sleeping in bus stations several times when he could not find somewhere to stay."[29]

Though the cause of death was a heart attack, Omalu was curious about the earlier diagnosis of Webster's brain damage. Omalu removed the brain and noted how normal it appeared. Just to be sure, he obtained permission to examine the brain in more detail. He made thin slices of the brain and sent them off to a laboratory to be stained. The stain, he knew, could highlight particular proteins found in the brains of Alzheimer's patients and boxers suffering from CTE.

Tau Tangles

When viewed under his microscope, Omalu saw tau proteins, a sure sign of CTE. The tau protein is one of the substances that make up nerve tissues. When the brain is concussed, or shaken, nerve fibers become torn, and the tau protein is released, forming a kind of sludge.

The brain attempts to clean up the tau protein, and if allowed to rest for a long time, it can usually accomplish that task. However, if the jolts and hits continue, the tau spillage becomes more profound and too much for the brain to handle. The abnormally high amounts of the protein form what look like brownish tangles in the brain tissue. The tau tangles interfere with communication within the brain—eventually killing off brain cells.

> **tau**
>
> A protein found in brain cells that is released when the brain is damaged by the jarring that takes place during a concussion.

Scientists know that in the case of an Alzheimer's patient, the tau tangles begin in the hippocampus, a deep part of the brain. Webster's hippocampus showed no tau tangles, so it was clear he did not have Alzheimer's disease. In CTE the tau tangles originate in the cortex, the large outer part of the brain. Inspection of Webster's cortex revealed the presence of the tau. For the first time, a football player was found to have CTE, previously believed to strike only boxers who had taken too many blows to the head. More important, this was evidence that over time a history of concussions could have disastrous results for an athlete.

Omalu also performed autopsies on other retired athletes who died, including Andre Waters of the Philadelphia Eagles and Terry Long of the Pittsburgh Steelers, both of whom had exhibited symptoms of CTE after retirement. Their symptoms included anger problems, depression, and mental confusion. Omalu's research found evidence of CTE in their brains, too.

How Soon Can Athletes Return?

While research into the brains of athletes and CTE continues, other research has focused on preventing young athletes from having the same

Help from Woodpeckers?

A recent study that may reveal new information about concussions is focused on woodpeckers. Scientists know that these birds hammer their beaks into tree trunks approximately 12,000 times per day at a speed of 15 miles per hour—all to find food within the wood. Researchers at Beihang University in Bejing, China, wondered how the birds avoid destroying their brains in the process.

First, the researchers used ultra-high-speed cameras to record the pecking motion and sensors to measure the force with which caged woodpeckers pecked. They found that the force of the woodpecker hammering measures as much as 1,000 g-force—10 times as much as the hits UNC researcher Kevin Guskiewicz was measuring on the football field. They also took scans of the birds' skulls and examined them at a microscopic level.

The results have initiated discussion among scientists about the need for a new type of protective helmet. The woodpecker's brain is packed tightly within the skull, which keeps it stable instead of sloshing around as a human brain does during a concussion. The woodpecker's inner skull is padded with spongy bone that can absorb shocks, too—both at the forehead and the back of the skull. "These findings would be applied to human protective devices such as sport helmet designs," says Yubo Fan, leader of the research team.

Quoted in *Toronto Star*, "Why Don't Woodpeckers Get Concussions?," October 27, 2011. www.thestar.com.

outcome. Not every bump or jolt to the head causes a concussion, and not every concussion is a career ender. Because of this ambiguity, some researchers have dedicated themselves to finding more reliable ways of telling whether an athlete has sustained a concussion, and if so, how long he or she should be sidelined.

In the early 1990s head-trauma specialist Mark Lovell and the Pittsburgh Steelers' team neurosurgeon Joseph Maroon decided to create a test to show when a concussed athlete could return to play. The result is known as Immediate Post-concussion Assessment and Cognitive Testing, or ImPACT. Before their season begins, athletes take what is called a baseline test, to determine the level of brain activity. The test addresses 21 different mental activities including thinking, memory, sight, and reaction speed.

The first use of the ImPACT test occurred in 1993. "Since it was before the boom in personal computers," explain Linda Carroll and David Roser in *The Concussion Crisis*, "Lovell had to rely on lengthy face-to-face interviews, standardized pencil and paper tests of memory and cognition, and a stopwatch to measure each player's reaction time."[30]

Today the ImPACT test is in the form of software and is usually administered to athletes by a doctor, trainer, nurse, or psychologist at the beginning of the season. When an athlete sustains a concussion, he or she takes the test again, and that score is compared with the baseline test. Doctors or trainers can monitor the athlete's recovery and use those results in deciding when to allow the athlete to return to playing.

However, the test has limitations. At least one athlete complained of symptoms—headaches, blurred vision, and fogginess—even though his ImPACT score indicated he could be cleared to resume playing. Others, including some professional athletes, have found a way to beat the ImPACT test. In order to keep from being sidelined at some point in the future, they purposely perform poorly on the baseline test. That way any deterioration of their speed or memory that shows up on the test after a concussion will not be so evident. NFL commissioner Roger Goodell admitted in 2011 that concussion-test cheating is "an issue the league needs to address."[31]

Data from Within the Helmet

Since collisions are intrinsic to the game of football, some research has concentrated on minimizing the damage to players. At the University of North Carolina, researcher Kevin Guskiewicz has focused some of his work on making the game of football safer. To do that, he wanted to see how many blows to the head the UNC players were getting during a season.

accelerometers

Sensors placed in football helmets that measure the force and number of hits to the brain sustained by a player.

To get an accurate count, Guskiewicz customized UNC players' helmets by embedding little sensors called accelerometers into their padding—at a cost of nearly $1,500 per helmet. The accelerometers measure and record not only the number of hits players get to their heads but also the location and force of those hits. That data is instantly relayed to a computer on the sideline during games or in the training room at practice.

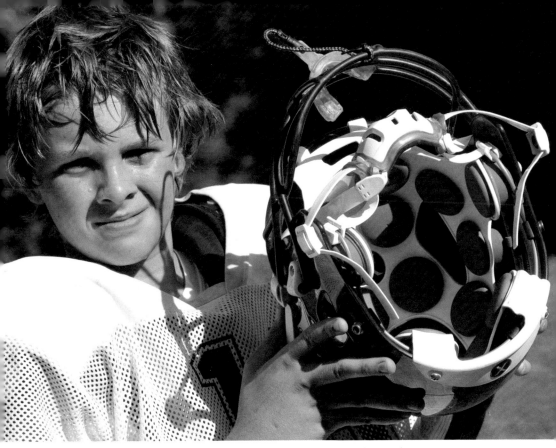

Helmets with special sensors, such as the one displayed here by a Maryland middle school quarterback, measure a baseline level of brain activity at the beginning of the season. Baseline measurements can help doctors determine when an athlete is fully recovered from a concussion.

The unit of measurement Guskiewicz uses is g-force, short for gravitational force. *Time* magazine reporter Jeffrey Kluger puts the g-force data collected by the accelerometers into perspective: "Liftoff of a Saturn V moon rocket exposed its crew to a maximum of four g's. A roller coaster may exceed six g's. College football players, by contrast, collide with each other with an impact of nearly 23 g's—and that's the average. Higher-end blows range from 85 to 100 g's."[32] According to Guskiewicz, the highest hit he has recorded so far in his UNC experiments was 180 g's.

The number of hits was as astounding as the force of the hits. In practices and games combined, some players were taking as many as 1,000 hits to the head over the course of a football season. Guskiewicz terms the hits "sub-concussive" because none of those hits is enough to cause a concussion. However, that many hits each year over a college career—and likely thousands more if the the player were to extend his career by turning pro—could produce a cumulative effect that might very well endanger that player.

Playing Safer

Guskiewicz's accelerometer data has proved to be helpful in teaching UNC players safer methods of blocking and tackling, too. When the accelerometers show that one of the players is taking too many jolts to one part of his helmet, Guskiewicz can set up the video of the practice or game and synchronize the data and video feed to see exactly what was happening during those hits.

In one instance, he took a player aside, pointing out that his accelerometers were recording dangerous hits. Guskiewicz was concerned by the large number of hits the accelerometers were recording at the top of the player's helmet—12 in one game. He pointed to the video, which clearly showed the player dropping his head to make the tackle using the top of his helmet—a stance that could lead to serious injury to the player being tackled and a concussion to the player doing the tackling.

Knowing this, young players today are taught instead to lead into a tackle with the shoulder. By pinpointing such moments, Guskiewicz is trying to reinforce safer ways of playing football.

Continuing Concussion Research

Concussion research in the twenty-first century is ongoing—fueled in part by the very visible declines and deaths of well-known athletes. In 2011, for instance, 28-year-old professional hockey player Derek Boogaard died of a drug overdose. Boogaard was known as an enforcer, a player who is more valuable for his fighting prowess on the ice than for scoring goals. Boogaard had suffered scores of concussions and blows to the head from fighting throughout his time in Canadian youth leagues and the NHL.

When his brain was autopsied, it was clear that Boogaard had suffered from CTE. Researchers were shocked; they had never seen such evidence of CTE in a person so young. Had he lived, Boogaard's parents were told, he would have had severe dementia by the time he was middle-aged. Ann McKee, the director of the brain bank at Boston University's Center for the Study of Traumatic Encephalopathy, performed the autopsy. "That surprised me," she admitted. "To see this amount [of the brown tau spots]? That's a wow moment."[33]

Concussion research has been boosted by growing support of NFL and NHL players who have made pledges to help concussion research in the most personal way. As of December 2011, more than 500 current and former athletes had agreed to donate their brains to scientific research. Perhaps, say scientists, the information gleaned from those brains, as well as other research, can make all athletes safer.

"I keep telling kids, Your brain is not your knee. It's not your shoulder. It's your future," says Gerard Gioia of the Center for Neuroscience Research in Washington, DC. "We have to protect it better than we are."[34]

Overuse Injuries

In 2011, 38-year-old Minneapolis cyclist Donald Neally was diagnosed with hyperextension of the neck. He had never heard of that condition before but learned quickly that neck hyperextension is not an uncommon problem with people who ride their bikes on a regular basis. "It was explained to me this way: When you ride, your position is to lean forward and bent over, to minimize the resistance and go faster," Neally says. "But what got me into trouble was that I had my handlebars set too low for my body. I'm six foot three, and I'd been leaning too far down, which put a lot of my weight forward, putting pressure on my neck muscles."[35]

Neally's doctor called his hyperextended neck an overuse injury, meaning that over time his positioning on the bike caused his neck muscles to spasm—painfully. The doctor advised Neally to refrain from riding for a week or two. After that, he could go back to riding, starting with just a few miles and gradually increasing the distance. Neally also raised the handlebars on his bike so his shoulder, arms, and neck would not be in the position of bearing the weight of his body as he rode. He followed his doctor's advice, and after a few weeks his neck problems went away.

Overuse injuries are a common reason that athletes—whether amateurs or professionals—consult sports medicine specialists. These painful injuries are the result of repetitive stress over time. Most frequently they affect muscles, tendons, and joints. According to the American Orthopaedic Society for Sports Medicine, doctors are noticing a trend in which the numbers of patients suffering from overuse injuries is increasing and the average age of those patients is dropping. In 2010 the CDC reported that high school athletes alone accounted for 500,000 office visits—most of them due to overuse injuries.

Many of these injuries can be treated by adjusting workout routines and resting to allow the injury to heal. However, sometimes rest and adjustments to routine are not enough. Sports medicine specialists have looked to new research to find ways to relieve pain resulting from overuse injuries as well as minimize the recovery time after sustaining such an injury. Some of this research occurs by testing, experimentation, and analysis in laboratories. In at least one case, an operating room and a major-league pitching mound provided the laboratory for a sports medicine breakthrough.

Pitchers and Elbows

The problem orthopedic surgeon Frank Jobe, the Los Angeles Dodgers' team physician, hoped to solve in 1974 was that of an overuse injury—one of the most devastating incurred by baseball pitchers. It is the injury to an important part of the elbow called the ulnar collateral ligament, or UCL. The UCL is a tough band of tissue that helps bind the large upper bone in the upper arm, the humerus, to the two bones in the forearm.

> **ulnar collateral ligament**
>
> The band of connective tissue binding the large bone in the upper arm to the two bones in the forearm.

Elite women cyclists compete in an international championship race. Avid and competitive cyclists often suffer from neck hyperextension, a painful overuse injury that results from the forward-leaning position common to the sport.

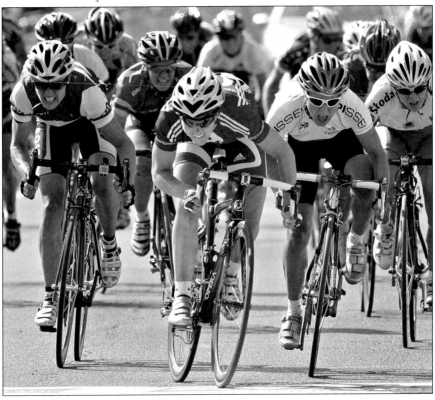

The repetitive motion of throwing a baseball in addition to the speed of the throw, puts a great deal of strain on the UCL—especially when the pitcher throws hard. UCL stress is one of the main reasons baseball managers keep a pitch count, to make sure the pitcher is not endangering that ligament by throwing too many pitches in one outing and damaging the UCL. Occasionally, the UCL will stretch, becoming weaker and making it difficult for the pitcher to throw with any intensity. A far more serious injury is when the UCL finally ruptures, or pops.

Until the mid-1970s, a UCL injury—either a sprain or a complete rupture—signaled the end of a pitcher's career. Though he might be able to throw, he would not be able to put enough spin or speed on the ball to be effective. One famous victim of a UCL injury was Sandy Koufax, whose brilliant career as a pitcher for the Los Angeles Dodgers was shortened in 1966 by what was then simply called "dead arm." The forced retirement of talented pitchers such as Koufax was disappointing to fans, a hardship to the teams that depended on them, and most of all, devastating for the athletes themselves.

That changed in 1974, when Jobe met with All-Star pitcher Tommy John. John, who had severe elbow damage, would become the first ever to have an experimental surgery on his UCL—a surgery that made it possible for John to continue his Major League career for another 14 years.

An Experimental Procedure

Jobe met with John to discuss his upcoming retirement from baseball due to his chronically sore UCL. On Jobe's advice, John had taken time off from throwing and had gradually begun a regimen of strengthening exercises for his arm. Though he had made some progress, it was clear to Jobe that John had hit a plateau. "He did pretty well," Jobe remembers. "He worked hard, he got to the point where he could throw, but he couldn't really put anything on the ball beyond about 75 percent. So in that case, chances are, he wouldn't be able to get anybody out."[36]

At the time, no surgical options existed. But as the two talked, Jobe mentioned an idea he had had for a while. He believed it might be possible to replace a damaged UCL with a tendon from elsewhere in the body. Tendons and ligaments are very similar; a ligament attaches a bone to another bone, while a tendon attaches a muscle to a bone. Jobe knew that tendon transplants had been done on some polio patients in the

⚛ Running Faster, for a Shorter Distance

Runners frequently complain of overuse injuries—especially those that affect the knees, shins, and hips. A study described in the June 2011 edition of the *Journal of Strength and Conditioning Research* found that long-distance runners may be able to avoid many of those injuries by running faster for shorter distances. It was previously believed that overuse injuries were caused by the speed and intensity of the runs; however, that belief seemed to be contradicted by this new research.

In the study, led by John P. Abt, associate professor of sports medicine and nutrition at the University of Pittsburgh, scientists studied 12 competitive male and female long-distance runners to see how they responded to brief, high-intensity runs on a treadmill. All the athletes ran at approximately 95 percent of their maximum heart rate until they were exhausted. The average time it took for a runner to get to a state of exhaustion was about 18 minutes.

The researchers looked carefully at changes in shock absorption and joint motion as the athletes ran. Previous research suggests that running fatigue leads to altered joint motion and impact and that this may contribute to overuse injuries in long-distance runners. However, in this study, the fatigue associated with the shorter, faster runs did not lead to the joint pain experienced by those running a longer amount of time. If that is the case, runners may be able to get the same benefits of exercise with a much lower risk of overuse injuries by running for briefer periods at a faster rate.

1960s to strengthen an ankle or other joint that was weak from the effects of the disease.

Jobe told John that it was just an idea and made it clear that he did not know if the transplant would work with a UCL. He gave John an honest opinion of the likelihood of success—only about 1 percent. "I thought I could do the surgery," he recalls, "but would it hold up under the stress of throwing? That was the problem. We didn't know whether it would work or not. That's why I didn't give him a very good prognosis."[37]

Despite the uncertainty of whether the procedure would succeed, John was eager to try. "The thing that made it easy for me to say yes, let's have it, was when Dr. Jobe told me, 'You do not have to have the surgery, but if you don't, you'll never pitch in major league baseball again, as you know it,'" he says. "And I wanted to play baseball in the worst possible way. . . . Even a 1 percent chance was better than zero chance."[38]

Success

The surgery took about three hours. Jobe took a tendon, the palmarus longus, from the left-handed pitcher's right forearm. This tendon is not crucial to the athlete; in fact, about 15 percent of people do not even have this tendon in their forearm. After removing John's damaged ligament and moving the large ulnar nerve out of the way, Jobe drilled tunnels through the two bones, the ulna and the humerus. He then laced the bones together with the tendon in a figure-eight pattern.

palmarus longus

The tendon harvested from a pitcher's opposite forearm to replace the damaged UCL during Tommy John surgery.

Scientists say that the body eventually trains the tendon for its new role by supplying it with blood vessels that give it a good blood supply so it can "learn" to become a ligament. Researchers today still do not understand how this transformation occurs, but the surgery has proven successful in numerous cases. Jobe's groundbreaking procedure, now known as Tommy John surgery, was a complete success. After his year-long rehabilitation, John felt as if he could throw the ball as well as he ever had, and over the next 14 years won an additional 164 games. Today one in nine Major League pitchers owes his career to Tommy John surgery. The value of Jobe's surgery is especially evident by the fact that many players and managers have seriously proposed that Jobe be inducted into baseball's Hall of Fame—a first for any scientist.

Arthroscopy

Scientists have developed other surgical techniques—or have improved older ones—to help athletes recover from overuse injuries. Knee problems, for example, are a common overuse injury—especially in sports such as soccer, football, tennis, and skiing. For years the primary method of repairing damaged ligaments of the knee was highly invasive, requiring large incisions first to view the problem and then to fix it. Large incisions not only meant extensive scarring and a longer recuperation time but also presented a risk of infection.

Arthroscopic surgery, which became widely used in the 1960s, offers a way to address the problems and risks that can occur with traditional surgery. The surgeon uses a tiny camera-like optical instrument, called an arthroscope, which is attached to a thin tube. In arthroscopic knee surgery, for example, the tube is inserted into the joint via a tiny incision about the size of a small buttonhole. Once the damaged tendon has been examined, the surgeon makes one or two more small incisions and inserts other thin tubes onto which tiny surgical instruments are attached.

Using arthroscopy, an orthopedic surgeon examines the inside of a patient's knee for injury. The view from inside the joint appears on a screen (upper left). The development of arthroscopic surgery gave doctors a less-invasive treatment than traditional surgery for repairing tears and other overuse injuries.

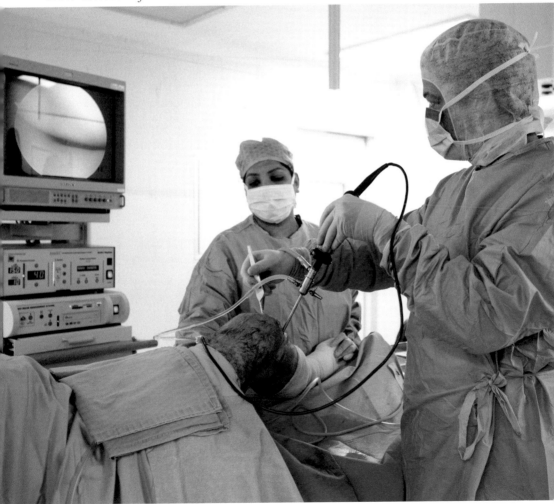

Tommy John Surgery in the Twenty-First Century

Since 1974, when Frank Jobe pioneered the ulnar collateral ligament (UCL) surgery named after his first patient, pitcher Tommy John, sports medicine researchers have become concerned about the numbers and ages of athletes seeking the surgery. In the late 1990s, only 12 percent of the patients were age 18 or younger. However, by 2005 that age group made up 33 percent of Tommy John patients.

Arthroscopy specialist E. Lyle Cain, fellowship director for the American Sports Medicine Institute in Birmingham, Alabama, feels that this increase is worrisome. "The reality is that this surgery is successful and that's good. But a disturbing trend of younger kids needing the surgery is troubling. This should be a wake-up call to parents and coaches that specialization in baseball where kids don't get adequate time off is very dangerous."

Cain cites reasons for the growing number of UCL injuries in teens, such as year-round baseball in warm-weather states and young pitchers throwing too hard for too many innings. He and others worry that young players are not doing enough conditioning and strength training to prevent UCL damage and instead see Tommy John surgery as a safety net. "It's great that the surgery is successful," he says, "but the prevention of the injury should be the goal. Kids should be urged to rest and be careful about saving their arms, rather than leading to long term problems at a young age."

Quoted in ScienceDaily, "'Tommy John' Surgery for Elbow Reconstruction Effective, but Number of Baseball Players Requiring It Alarming," July 12, 2008. www.sciencedaily.com.

By viewing the image sent from the arthroscope to a television monitor, the surgeon can do the repair. Arthroscopy has been hailed as one of the top three medical advances of the twentieth century.

According to technology analyst James Laskaris, research by Hinsdale (Illinois) Orthopedics Associates released in June 2011 verified the advantages of arthroscopic surgery over traditional surgery. Because doctors most often use local anesthetic in arthroscopic surgery, patients can go home on the same day and immediately begin their recuperation. The data also found that arthroscopic surgery is less costly than traditional surgery. Arthroscopic hip surgery in the United States, for example, averages between $2,000 and $3,000, while traditional surgery ranges from $7,000 to $16,000.

Improved outcome is another reason that more patients opt for arthroscopic surgery. The Hinsdale study used a testing method known as the Harris Hip Scores to compare the results of arthroscopic and traditional hip surgery. The Harris Hip Score test is a patient questionnaire commonly used to evaluate the success of hip surgery. By asking surgery patients detailed questions about the amount and severity of pain, their range of motion after surgery, and recovery time, doctors hoped to learn how the two types of surgery compare. The study found that arthroscopic surgery patients averaged improvement of 26.4 percent compared with 20.5 percent for those who underwent traditional hip surgery. In addition, the study found that there were almost 80 percent fewer complications with arthroscopic hip surgery.

ACLs and Bone Structure

Some medical research addresses the reasons for sports-related injuries, to see if some way might be found to prevent those injuries from occurring. Especially devastating to an athlete is the painful tear of the anterior cruciate ligament, or ACL. Of the four main ligaments in the knee, the ACL is the most important factor in keeping the knee joint stable. It is the ACL, for instance, that allows a football running back to make quick cuts to change directions and avoid a tackle. Approximately 300,000 ACL injuries occur each year in the United States, and almost all of these are suffered by athletes.

anterior cruciate ligament

An important ligament that holds the knee in place.

Tarek O. Souryal, medical researcher and head physician for the NBA's Dallas Mavericks, has long been interested in the prevalence of ACL injuries. He recalls asking one of his professors years ago how common it was for an athlete to have ACL tears in both knees. To get an answer to his question, in the 1990s Souryal helped organize a survey of 1,100 athletes ranging in age from 15 to 60, who had torn an ACL.

"When we contacted those athletes, we were interested in learning how many had blown out their other knee, as well," Souryal says. "We found that 4 percent of those surveyed had blown out both ACLs. But we found something—actually two things that the athletes in this 4 percent group had in common. First, all of them were between ages 16 and 17. And the other thing is, every one of their X-rays looked funny."[39]

Research Helps Explain ACL Injuries

The oddity in those X-rays had to do with the notch, or tunnel-like part of the bone in which the ACL is found. "The ACL and posterior cruciate ligament (PCL) live in a tunnel at the end of your thigh bone," Souryal explains. "If that tunnel is very narrow (which you can detect by x-ray), then there's no room for the ACL to maneuver."[40]

In the study, all of the athletes who had torn both ACLs had the narrow notch. This was the first study to suggest a possible link between bone structure and the likelihood of injuring the ACL. But the research did not end there. "What followed my original question," Souryal says, "is the classic example of research—you often find out way more than you expected to know. And that leads to more questions."[41]

To test their theory that the narrow notch at the end of the thigh bone contributed to ACL tears, Souryal and his team undertook a massive project of x-raying the knees of 1,000 high school athletes, and following them for the next two years. "Whenever a player went down with an ACL injury," he says, "we looked at his notch. And it was phenomenal: The kids who were blowing out their ACLs all had those narrow notches. We stopped the study early because the numbers were so dramatic."[42]

Again, the research led to more questions. Knowing about the link between the size of the ACL notch and the likelihood of an ACL injury, says Souryal, made them wonder about the possibility of preventing the injury for those who have smaller ACL notches. At the time, Souryal wondered:

> The biggest question right now is, what lives inside the narrow notch? Does a small ACL live in a narrow notch and tears because it's never had the room to grow properly? Or does a normal-sized ACL live in the small notch and rupture because it doesn't have the room? . . . If it is a normal sized ACL in the notch, then maybe we can go in there surgically and widen the notch, and perhaps save that person from an ACL rupture.[43]

Sometimes research is thwarted by the lack of powerful technology, and that was the case in the early 1990s. MRIs were not yet sophisticated enough to provide a clear image of the notches and the ACLs in the knees.

Several years later, however, MRIs had become far clearer, and Souryal and his team at last had an answer to their question. The ACLs within the small notches were small, and those ACLs in the normal-sized notches were normal. Preventive surgery would not help athletes avoid an ACL tear. "I guess the next unanswered question is, 'What causes the size of notches?'" Souryal speculates today. "Maybe genetic? That's the next question."[44]

Platelet-Rich Plasma

New research has resulted in improved surgical methods as well as a better understanding of ligaments, tendons, and joints. However, many doctors are excited about a new procedure that may make some surgeries unnecessary—or hasten recovery after surgery. It is called platelet-rich plasma (PRP) therapy, and it takes advantage of the body's natural powers to speed healing after an injury.

For decades, scientists have known about the healing powers of the platelets in blood. Platelets are colorless, irregularly shaped discs that are present in blood. They are not cells but rather fragments of cells. When a person is injured, platelets

platelets

Fragments of cells found in blood that help speed healing and blood clotting.

gather at the site of the injury; their sticky surface allows them to adhere to the edges of the wound and release chemicals that start the process of blood clotting. The chemicals in platelets also contain hormones that speed cell regrowth.

In the 1990s scientists began experimenting with the idea of injecting concentrated platelets into the site of an injury or surgical wound to speed up the healing. The process involves taking some blood from the athlete and spinning it rapidly in a machine called a centrifuge. The spinning separates the plasma with its platelets from the rest of the blood. The concentrated platelets are then injected back into the athlete's injury.

"The first doctors to get on board with platelet-rich plasma were oral surgeons and plastic surgeons," says osteopathic physician Joseph Aiello, "because . . . they saw an enhanced healing when they were doing re-constructive surgery in the bones, and plastic surgeons when they were doing facial surgeries, and they started using the platelet-rich plasma to enhance the healing of those surgeries."[45]

Promising Research

Since then, scores of other physicians have used PRP therapy to help professional athletes recover from surgery and from sore, inflamed joints and muscles. Tiger Woods had PRP therapy to help speed his recovery from ACL surgery in 2009. That same year, Pittsburgh Steelers wide receiver Hines Ward had PRP therapy to speed his recovery from a sprained knee so that he could play in the Super Bowl. In 2011 Kobe Bryant of the Los Angeles Lakers had the procedure done on his chronically sore right knee.

More and more athletes have sought PRP therapy, often based on the good outcomes of their teammates. Doctors have been optimistic about the therapy, saying that because the athlete is receiving his or her own blood, there are virtually no risks of infection. "Nobody knows just what injuries respond to platelets," says David Altcheck, orthopedic surgeon and medical director for the New York Mets baseball team. "There's a very good case for tennis elbow, and we know if you cut yourself with a razor, platelets work [by clotting]. But there are no side effects. It's as safe as medical treatments come."[46]

In 2012 the Mayo Clinic released the results of a study on a combination of PRP therapy and tenotomy—a process of repeated needle-sticks (pokes with a surgical needle) to break up scar tissue in an injured tendon. Many physicians believe that tenotomy prompts the body's own cells to start the rebuilding process, just as concentrated platelets in PRP therapy are believed to do.

The study included 34 patients with long-standing injuries of tendons and other soft tissues within the body. In the first stage of the study, researchers used ultrasound to guide a needle to the injured area. The physician repeatedly poked the tendon with the needle, causing minor bleeding within the tissue. After that, the patients were injected with platelets from their own blood.

The results were promising. According to researchers, more than 70 percent of the patients had better use of their tendons, and 76 percent reported less pain. Even so, experts insist that this was just one study. "Larger studies are still necessary to determine whether the combination is particularly helpful for certain injuries or types of tendons,"[47] says researcher Jay Smith, the author of the study.

Doctors throughout the United States have had good results with PRP therapy. They see it as more than a procedure for the likes of Tiger Woods and Kobe Bryant. "It's not just the professional athlete who needs to get back to their game," says PRP researcher Allan Mishra of Stanford University Medical Center. "Everyone wants to get back to what they do for play or work."[48]

Prosthetics Research

For Texas native Scott Odom, life had always circled around sports, especially basketball. His dream was to play in the NBA—a dream he believed he would achieve. "I had it all planned out," he remembers. "I was going to play in high school, get a scholarship, and go in the [NBA] draft. I know every kid says that, but I was that good, and was going to do it."[49]

In August 2011 he was showcasing his basketball talent in a three-on-three tournament in Los Angeles, when he received an invitation. The owner of the Texas Legends, the minor league basketball team affiliated with the NBA's Dallas Mavericks, invited him to try out for his team. Odom, 26, was elated. For any young basketball player, an opportunity to try out for an elite team such as the Legends would be an amazing accomplishment. For Odom, it was even more special. Odom lost his right leg to cancer at the age of 14. He now wears a prosthetic leg. And although he did not make the team, he still plays basketball with the same skill and fervor as many of his sound-bodied peers.

Athletes Missing Limbs

A prosthesis is an artificial limb or other body part to replace one that has been lost due to injury or disease. In Odom's case, the cause was bone cancer, discovered in an MRI on the first day of his freshman year of high school. Part of his leg was amputated, and after months of chemotherapy and a second operation the surgeons had to cut even higher.

For Canadian teen Lily Lange, it was a boating accident that tore off most of her right arm when she was five years old. "I had run out into the water to get in the boat,"[50] says Lange, now 17:

> My uncle was driving, and he'd just come back from taking my two older sisters for a ride. I wanted to go next, but he didn't even know I was [in the water]. I tripped and fell near the back of the boat, and my arm came in contact with the propeller. I don't

remember too much, which is probably a good thing because it was so traumatic. But now that arm ends at just under my elbow. I wear a prosthetic arm almost all the time—I'm so used to it, I don't really think about it anymore. I like to swim, run—pretty much anything I want to do.[51]

According to data released in 2011 by the Amputee Coalition, approximately 185,000 entire- or partial-limb amputations occur in the United States each year. The vast majority of those amputees are later fitted with a prosthesis to help them regain some of the function that their lost limb provided. Modern prosthetics research has also made it possible for amputees to ski, swim, cycle, do gymnastics, play basketball, and take part in a wide range of other sports activities.

> **prosthesis**
>
> An artificial limb or organ that replaces one damaged by injury or disease.

Prosthetic Technology Through the Ages

The use of prosthetics has a long history. In 2000, archaeologists discovered a tomb near the ancient Egyptian city of Thebes. They found the mummified remains of a 50- to 60-year-old woman with an artificial big toe attached to her right foot. Made of leather and wood, the toe was jointed in three places. Based on artifacts that were found in the mummy's burial chamber, archaeologists estimated that the remains date from between 1069 and 664 BC, making it the oldest prosthesis ever discovered.

During Europe's Middle Ages, roughly between AD 1000 and 1400, a knight who lost a hand or foot to an enemy's sword in battle relied on a prosthesis to continue his career. Blacksmiths, who also made knights' armor, created prostheses by hammering metal plates onto a wooden core that had been whittled into the same size and shape as the missing part. Using leather straps, the new appendage could then be fastened to the stump of the limb. Making the new hand appear lifelike was of little concern, for it was usually covered with a glove. Historians say that the glove's purpose was to hide an injury that revealed a knight's weakness.

In the early sixteenth century, a doctor in the French army, Ambroise Paré, invented both a hinged, mechanical hook-type hand and a prosthetic leg that featured a locking knee and a harness so the amputee could more easily put it on and take it off. In the late seventeenth century, a Dutch surgeon named Pieter Verduyn developed a prosthetic leg that could be attached to the body by a leather cuff. While these devices were definitely advances over the prostheses of the past, they were still undeniably bulky and very heavy, since they were made of wood, metal, and leather.

War Brings Innovation

Not surprisingly, wars throughout history have driven the quest for creating and improving new prostheses. After the Civil War, during which an estimated 60,000 to 70,000 soldiers had legs or arms amputated, prosthetics changed from a cottage industry, where they were made by hand by individuals, to an actual manufacturing industry. The factory-produced prostheses were not very different from those of a century before, but the materials had improved. The first use of rubber in constructing prosthetic hands in 1863 was a breakthrough because the texture was more like that of skin, and a hand made of rubber was more resilient than one made of wood and far less likely to break or chip.

Improvements continued in the 1940s, as a flood of amputees returned after World War II. The US government put millions of dollars into research to develop new prostheses, made lighter by the use of plastics and aluminum, as well as new methods to fit them to the returning veterans. At the time, the emphasis was on cosmetics—making the artificial limbs look as realistic as possible.

"It was form over function," says Wisconsin native Eileen Malek, whose father lost a leg in the Korean War. "But the idea of a leg that let him play sports wouldn't have occurred to him. And if it had, Dad wouldn't have wanted one. All he cared about was that both pant legs were filled out, and he could walk without crutches so no one could tell he was missing his leg."[52]

Attitudes since that time have changed, and as a result, so have the prostheses. "We just steadily advanced on some of the lessons learned from all the way back to the Civil War,"[53] says one Minneapolis prosthetist:

> For upper limbs, we got into body-controlled prosthetics, where you'd have to wear a harness around your back—you move your shoulder a certain way, and that makes a cable, like a bicycle cable, open or close the hand. Innovation just took off from there.

And instead of slowing down, the innovation has increased because of the wars now in Iraq and Afghanistan. You've got a surge in amputations because of the large number of IEDs [improvised explosive devices, or roadside bombs] frequently being used by the enemy. We're into electronics, microchips—virtually a whole new generation of prostheses is emerging from that."[54]

A disabled World War II veteran is fitted with an artificial leg in 1943. The return of thousands of servicemen with amputated limbs following the war prompted the federal government to spend millions of dollars on research to develop new prostheses.

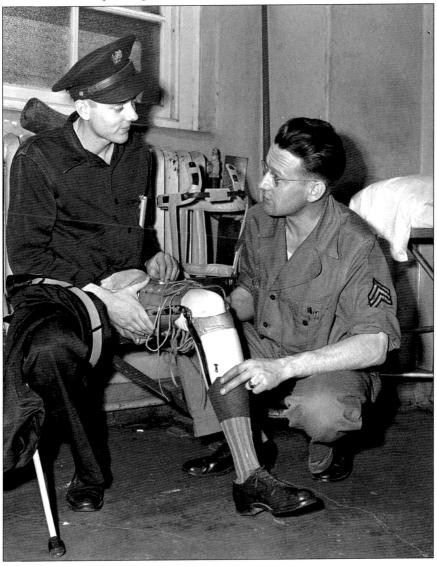

Designing a Custom Racing Bike

Years after the accident that cost him both of his arms, Hector Picard decided he would take part in a triathlon. He knew the running part of the event would be no problem, and he was confident that he could do the swimming on his back. The biking part, however, would be difficult. How could he ride a racing bike at a speed of 30 miles per hour (48 kph) and be able to brake and shift gears without hands? Picard tackled the problem himself.

"I bought a $100 Huffy, and some stuff at the hardware store, and I ended up using it for my first 10 triathlons. It was a lot harder because I couldn't change gears, so I kept it on the hardest gear to maximize the speed. I couldn't use the handbrakes, so I rerouted the handbrakes to the frame, so I can use my knees to hit the brakes."

Eventually the Signature Cycle Company helped by providing a custom bike, using some of Picard's ideas. When he competes, he does not use his prosthesis but puts his stump into a plumbing device called a coupler. That way, he can use his stump to push the buttons that change gears. "That's how I control the bike. I just move slightly, to hit the button," Picard says. "I think I have 28 gear selections. There are two switches, with two buttons on each. My stump is kind of pointy, so pushing the buttons isn't that hard."

Hector Picard, telephone interview by author, February 10, 2012.

Myoelectrics

One of the most useful ideas in modern prosthetics, myoelectrics, was introduced in 1955. Continued research has led to more sophisticated prosthetics. Myoelectrics is based on the idea that muscles generate electrical impulses in the body. Electrodes are placed inside a prosthetic arm and fit to the wearer so they are very close to the skin over certain muscles. When the wearer flexes that muscle, the electrodes respond by opening or closing the prosthetic hand. That allows the wearer to grasp

myoelectrics

The use of the electrical impulses created by a muscle to control the movement or operation of a prosthetic device.

a pool cue, hold on to a bike's handlebars, and a range of other activity-related movements.

Becky Born, a prosthetist with Shriner's Hospital in Minneapolis, demonstrates a myoelectric arm built for a young girl whose hand was amputated after a lawn mower accident—one of the most common reasons for childhood amputations. "It's a fairly simple process to learn,"[55] says Born:

> She'll control the hand opening or closing by moving a muscle in her arm. She doesn't have a hand, but she has her forearm. If she flexes the inner muscle of the forearm, the electrode inside the prosthesis that is right on that muscle picks up the electric current and that powers the mechanism that will open the hand. So then, when she flexes the muscle on the outer part of her forearm, that will close the hand. It's really, really important that arm fits very snug, right against the skin, so the electrodes can work the way they're supposed to.[56]

Sport-Specific Limbs

While prosthetic arms and legs are important for an amputee to become more active, some prostheses used by athletes today are very sports-specific, meaning they are intended for one particular sport. One such device tested by researchers at the University of South Florida in 2010 is a prosthetic arm made especially for a golfer. It does not resemble an arm at all but rather is a 6–inch (15-cm) piece of polyurethane that can be screwed into the socket of an existing prosthesis. This type of prosthesis is known as a terminal device, or TD.

> **terminal device**
>
> A specialized attachment screwed into the socket of a prosthesis that allows the wearer to play a sport like tennis or golf.

This particular TD, made by the amputee sporting equipment source TRS, is called the Eagle Golf TD. It is designed to slide over the shaft of a golf club, and then to jam into place on the grip of the club. Researchers wanted to know how well their device worked and whether it was hard or easy to learn to control. They also wanted to know whether an amputee using the device would feel comfortable playing golf with sound-bodied friends. Researcher Jason Highsmith, assistant professor in the University of South Florida's School of Physical Therapy and Rehabilitation Science, needed to know whether an amputee without golf experience could "muster a reasonable swing sufficient to enjoy recreational participation in golf."[57]

Alan Hines, who agreed to participate in the study, was pleasantly surprised at how quickly he learned to use the device and how well he could make contact with the ball. Hines, who had lost part of his right arm from an electrical accident 11 years before, was resigned to never playing any sport again. He admitted afterward that he had been doubtful he could use the device, since he had never played golf before his accident. After the test, he was excited about the prospect of playing golf with his 14-year-old son, although he was not hopeful about winning. "We'll have to play and see how bad he can beat me,"[58] he says.

Filling a Need

Not all research that helps amputees enjoy sports is the work of engineering or medical companies. Some ideas have come from amputees themselves. That is the case with a Florida man named Hector Picard, who lost both arms in an electrical accident.

A former electrician for a Florida power company, Picard had no interest in being sedentary, nor did he want to be defined by the fact that he has no arms. Picard was fitted with a prosthesis for his left arm, but because of the severe burns he had suffered on his chest, he could not support a prosthesis for his right arm.

He found that the available sports prostheses were designed for one-arm amputees who could use their remaining arm to do most of the work shooting and catching a ball. So to enable himself to play basketball, he developed his own prosthetic attachment that allowed him to catch the ball as well as shoot it. "I just used a plain old plastic bucket," he says. "I cut it up, used nuts and bolts to attach it to the prosthesis on my left arm. It worked great—I used it forever. It was definitely a good head-turner at the park. People would stop just to watch me play basketball."[59]

To coach and train his daughter's Little League team, he devised a way to attach an aluminum bat to his prosthesis. By flicking a ball into the air with his left foot, he could hit grounders and fly balls to the girls for practice. At least one of his devices, the basketball prosthetic, was picked up by TRS. "Yeah, they saw what I could do with it, and they're going to start marketing it," says Picard. "It will be called the HP Hoopster."[60]

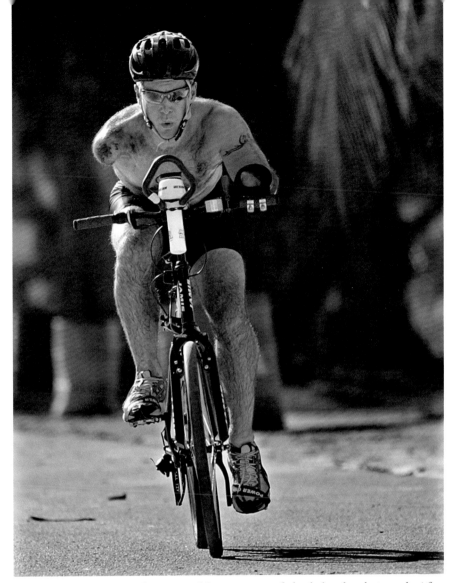

Hector Picard trains for a triathlon on one of the bikes he designed. After losing both of his arms in an electrical accident, Picard designed and built a custom racing bike for competitions. He also designed a prosthetic attachment that allowed him to catch and shoot a basketball.

The Flex-Foot

Picard is not the only sports-minded amputee who has designed new prostheses for athletes. Van Phillips of California lost his left leg below the knee as a result of a water-skiing accident in 1976. Soon afterward, he was measured for a prosthetic leg made from wood and rubber. An accomplished athlete before the accident, Phillips felt his new life was "like the sentence from hell."[61]

Katherine Bomkamp, Student Inventor

An estimated 80 percent of amputees suffer from phantom limb pain—the sensation of pain in a limb that is no longer there. A device called the Pain-Free Socket shows promise for eliminating these unpleasant sensations for athletes and others who have lost limbs to injury and illness.

Its inventor, Katherine Bomkamp, was in high school in 2007 when she came up with the idea. She had often accompanied her father, a disabled veteran, to Walter Reed Hospital in Washington, DC, for appointments, and often chatted with others in the waiting room. Amputees coming home from Iraq and Afghanistan complained about phantom limb pain—which doctors treated with painkillers and other addictive drugs. Bomkamp wondered about other treatment options. "My thought process was: When I pull a muscle, I apply heat to it. If I applied the same concept to treating phantom pain, I thought that would work."

For her high school science fair, 16-year-old Bomkamp created a prototype of her idea: a socket (the part of a prosthetic limb that touches the amputation site) with heated socks (like those used by hunters) as the heat source. She sought advice from engineers, prosthetists, and others. After making various adaptations—such as using more sophisticated electronics so that the amputee could control its temperature—she patented her invention. As of 2011 she is in talks with a prosthetic company about licensing the rights to sell her device. At age 18 Bomkamp was inducted into the National Gallery for America's Young Inventors.

Quoted in Nicole Laporte, "Don't Know How? Well, Find Someone Who Does," *New York Times*, November 11, 2011. www.nytimes.com.

Before the accident Phillips had been studying mass communications and advertising at Arizona State University. After the accident he changed his academic focus to prosthetics and orthotics. He later enrolled in Northwestern University's Biomedical Engineering program, where he began experimenting with a new kind of prosthetic leg. Very little had changed since World War II and the Korean War in terms of prosthetics, Phillips found. The legs available were cosmetically accurate but useless for an athlete.

Most of Phillips's research consisted of observing the way animals use and store energy. Explains *New York Times* reporter Carol Pogash, "[Phillips] studied ligaments that store muscle energy, observing the tendons of porpoises, kangaroos and cheetahs, noting how the cheetah's hind leg landed and compressed, and the elastic nature of it."[62] His aim was to design a prosthetic leg that would mimic this action. Phillips called his design Flex-Foot. It has a J-shaped blade that does the work of the leg muscles, flexing just as leg muscles would, and propelling the runner forward.

Phillips began building various Flex-Foot prostheses in his basement laboratory in the early 1980s. In 2000 he sold his designs to an Icelandic company, which continues to make and sell them. The response from Flex-Foot users has been overwhelming. Sarah Reinertsen, who lost a leg to a bone disorder at age 7, switched from her hollow wooden leg to a Flex-Foot when she was 12 years old. She says that when she first tried it, she felt as if she were "walking on a cloud."[63] In 2005, at age 30, Reinertsen became the first female amputee ever to complete Hawaii's famous Ironman triathlon.

Surgical Innovations

Although prosthesis designs have steadily improved over time, studies done in the early twenty-first century showed that even state-of-the-art limbs still had drawbacks. One of the biggest was difficulty of use. The other was discomfort.

A 2003 study by the Mayo Clinic in Rochester, Minnesota, found that only 47 percent of below-the-knee amputees successfully used their prostheses. The success rate was even more disappointing for above-the-knee amputees—only 13 percent. Those numbers, plus the disturbing prediction by researchers that the number of amputees in the United States was likely to double by 2030, created an urgency to solve the problems that were making prosthesis use difficult.

According to the study, there were two main reasons for the unsuccessful outcomes of prostheses. One was falls—an unfortunate part of learning to walk with a prosthetic leg. But sometimes falls can cause injuries to the sensitive tissue around the amputation site and make wearing

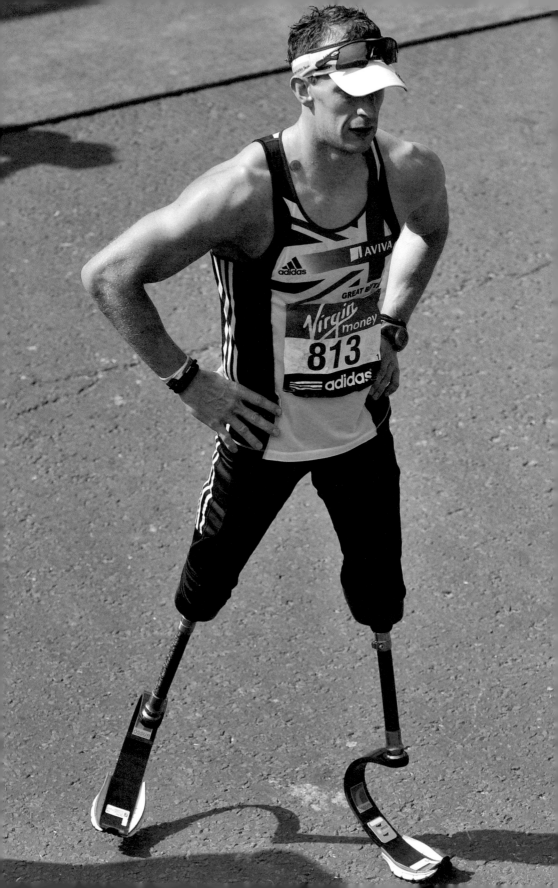

A runner with a pair of prosthetic blades reaches the finish line at a 2011 marathon in London. Prostheses have undergone many design changes over the years. The j-shaped blade flexes just as the leg muscles would and propels the runner forward.

the prosthesis uncomfortable. Another reason for the poor outcomes, experts believe, was the quality of amputation surgery.

Studies in the 1990s found that the most junior member of a surgical team is often the one who does the surgery. As a result, many amputees had to return to the hospital for additional surgery—usually in the first 6 months after receiving their prosthesis. Prosthetist Bill Copeland agrees, saying "We all, as prosthetists, see a lot of very bad amputations."[64]

Over time, surgeons have learned that the most successful amputations prepare the site for a future prosthetic limb by attaching muscles to bones, as well as retracting (moving back) the nerves. If nerves are left too close to the amputation site, they may come in contact with the prosthesis and cause pain. Studies have also revealed the importance of rounding off bones near the site to prevent sharp edges from irritating the stump, causing bleeding or infection. Researchers are confident that with better training and closer attention to such details, surgeons doing amputations can prevent much of the discomfort that keeps amputees from making full use of their prosthetics and engaging in active lifestyles.

Computerized Prosthetics

One of the most exciting innovations for amputees eager to become active again is known as CAREN, an acronym for computer-assisted rehabilitation environment. Invented by a medical technology company in the Netherlands and originally designed for use by the military, today CAREN is helping both military and civilian amputees reach their athletic potential.

CAREN is a virtual reality environment in which patients getting used to a new prosthesis can test themselves. Harvey Naranjo, the coordinator of the Military Advanced Training Center at Walter Reed Hospital, likens CAREN to "a Wii on crack."[65]

A patient wearing a new prosthetic leg walks on a treadmill that is mounted on a 5-foot-by-5-foot platform (1.5 m by 1.5 m). The platform moves up, down, right, left, forward, and backward. The treadmill requires the patient to keep moving as the platform adapts to what the user is doing and what sort of terrain he or she is moving through—whether moving down a busy city street, running in a forest, or even playing a video game in which the amputee is guiding a boat by using his or her feet.

"That's the one I tried," says one prosthetist. "I was eager to see what my patients would experience."[66]

> I was in total control of what I was doing—in this case, steering a boat by moving my feet. It's great in that you're in charge of your environment. You're in a harness, so you can't get hurt if you stumble or fall. I'm completely in control of the boat, as I look at the images on the screens around me—I step forward, the boat goes faster, step back, the boat slows down. Step right, the boat goes right; step left, it goes left. It's like I'm a big joystick.[67]

Cameras and other instruments constantly feed data about the patient's gate and stride to computers. This information helps doctors or occupational therapists determine whether a prosthesis needs even the slightest adjustment. The CAREN platform needs to be incredibly precise in reacting to the user's movements. In fact, one researcher notes that the CAREN platform can self-correct to balance a newly sharpened pencil on its point.

Research has resulted in state-of-the-art technology like CAREN, improved medical intervention before an athlete receives a prosthesis, and an ever-expanding array of new prosthetic limbs for different sports. As a result, more and more athletes with missing limbs will likely enjoy healthier, more active lives.

The Exciting Future of Sports Medicine

The strides made in medicine over the last 50 years have resulted in broader knowledge and an array of new technologies for diagnosing and treating sports injuries. Glimpses into the future of sports medicine show even more advances to come—advances that will almost certainly enable a new generation of athletes to reach their highest potential.

One of the most talked-about concerns in sports medicine is the frequency and severity of concussions among professional and amateur athletes. While researchers have learned a great deal about the causes and effects of these traumatic brain injuries, so far their studies have been limited by the nature of the work. The brain of a living person cannot be studied in the same depth as the brain of a person who has died. This has limited what scientists can learn about concussions in living athletes. "Concussion is global damage to the brain, and we have no machine to show that in a living person. That's one of the frustrations of brain study," says Michael K. Lee, a brain researcher at the University of Minnesota. "We know that just because symptoms of concussion are gone doesn't mean it is safe to resume playing. So there is a great deal of uncertainty—you go back too soon and you could be damaging the brain even further. We just don't know."[68]

New Types of MRI Show Promise

Some researchers are trying to improve diagnostic tools that will help doctors determine when it is safe for an athlete to return to play. The most promising methods could be a combination of two types of MRI technology—a functional MRI (fMRI) and diffusion tensor imaging (DTI) scans.

A standard MRI cannot see the microscopic changes a concussion causes within the brain. Rather than focusing on *seeing* such damage, an fMRI measures the abnormal changes in activity in the brain caused by concussion. "The fMRI looks at the amount of activity in the brain when

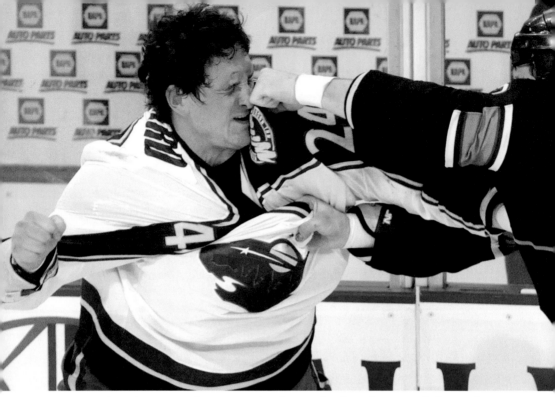

Hockey player Derek Boogaard is hit in the face during a fight on the ice in 2009. Boogaard, who died in 2011, suffered from a degenerative brain disorder caused by repeated blows to the head. The inability to fully study the brains of living athletes limits understanding of traumatic brain injuries like Boogaard's.

you do a particular task,"[69] explains Christophe Lenglet, assistant professor at the Center for Magnetic Resonance Research at the University of Minnesota.

> Iron in your red blood cells has magnetic properties, so we use that to measure on an MRI—to see how much blood is flowing through the brain when you're asked to do something. Increased flow of oxygen-rich blood [is associated with] increased brain activity. We could show you a series of pictures, for example, while you're lying in the MRI machine, and then ask you to remember them. So minutes later, while your brain works to recall the images you saw, we watch the screen to see the flow of blood—the activity—in that particular part of the brain. If we see that the flow of blood to that part of the brain is less than normal, that may indicate that the effects of the concussion are still there.[70]

The DTI Scan

Concussion researchers are even more excited about the DTI, another type of MRI. Rather than measuring the changes in how the brain functions, the DTI focuses on the actual wiring of the brain. Brain cells use a system of fibers to communicate with one another, much like a telephone network with millions of connections. This is known as the brain's "white matter."

When a concussion occurs, the result can be a tearing of those vital connections between cells, compromising the brain's ability to function. While the fMRI is programmed to show the flow of blood in the brain, the DTI responds to the water that is present in brain cells. A healthy neural network will show up on the DTI scan in bright colors. Dark patches in the network, however, can signal that the wiring has tears, which means the connective fibers may have been damaged.

> **diffusion tensor imaging**
>
> A type of brain scan that focuses on the wiring of the brain, to see whether there is any indication of concussion.

Researchers hope that their work with these two different types of MRIs can provide important data about differences in a concussed athlete's brain and can help doctors and trainers decide whether an athlete can safely resume playing. Lenglet says that in the future, athletes in sports in which concussions are common, such as football and hockey, may benefit from having a baseline DTI before the season begins. "That would be the ideal," he says. "Doctors could then compare a DTI after an athlete [who has suffered a concussion] has rested, with the baseline DTI. That could help determine if the brain has healed and the athlete could return to his or her sport."[71]

Stem Cells and Healing Injuries

Some medical experts predict that injured athletes might one day routinely benefit from treatments that rely on cells taken from their own bodies. Although still considered experimental, these cells, known as stem cells, are being used more and more in many areas of medicine, including the treatment of sports injuries.

Especially promising, scientists say, are mesenchymal stem cells, or MSCs, which appear to be particularly effective in healing bone and cartilage. These are immature cells that have not yet developed into a particular type of cell—a bone cell or a cartilage cell, for instance. Unlike controversial procedures that use stem cells from human embryos, the treatments athletes would receive would use their own stem cells, known as adult stem cells.

mesenchymal stem cell

A type of adult stem cell that may be valuable in speeding healing in bones and cartilage.

According to the Institute of Regenerative and Molecular Orthopedics, stem cells are known as "the repairmen"[72] of the body because they use the body's natural healing process to repair injured tissue. Many of the injuries that benefit from stem cell injections are in parts of the body lacking a good blood supply, such as shoulder, elbow, and knee joints. By injecting stem cells into these sites, doctors find that the injuries heal faster.

The stem cells used in healing today are extracted by needle from bone marrow and fat. After getting enough of the cells—usually about 2 ounces (60 cc)—the doctor injects them into the site of the injury, such as a torn muscle. According to orthopedist Richard C. Lehman of the US Center for Sports Medicine, some of the most impressive results have been in athletes who have undergone Tommy John surgery. After the surgery, the elbow joint can take a year to heal. However, with stem cell injections, he says, "players are throwing four months later and are at full strength by the sixth month."[73]

Promising Results from MSCs

Much of the research on MSCs is being done using animals. Scott Rodeo, an orthopedist and associate team physician for the New York Giants football team, has researched stem cell treatments in laboratory surgeries on rats. Stem cell treatments used in the reconstruction of ACL and shoulder muscles in rats have yielded positive results. "In each case, stem cells clearly have some beneficial role in inducing tissue regeneration."[74] he says.

In a study whose results were released in October 2011, the University of Medicine and Dentistry of New Jersey found evidence that MSC therapy may have an important role in treating and repairing injuries to the spinal cord. The scientists used human MSCs to prompt repair of spinal injuries in zebrafish. The zebrafish is useful in this type of research because it has some characteristics similar to the human body, in particular, the way it regenerates damaged tissue. In their findings researchers noted that "although mesenchymal stem cells are widely known to be used in replacing damaged tissue, these stem cells may also recruit endogenous [made within the body] cells to help accelerate the repair process."[75]

A colored 3-D diffusion tensor imaging, or DTI, scan shows bundles of white matter nerve fibers that transmit nerve signals between the regions of the brain and between the brain and spinal cord. This new type of imaging enables researchers to see tears that signal possible damage to those fibers.

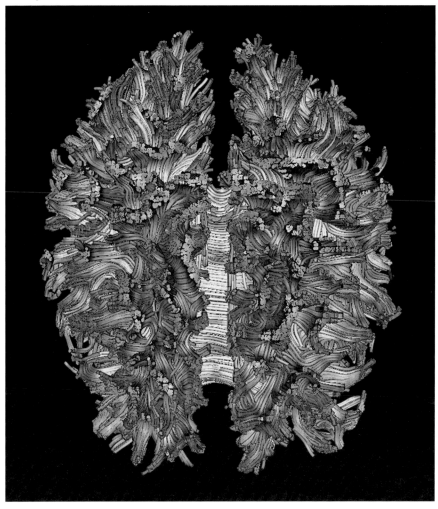

The Legacy of Albert Dow

All kinds of reasons drive a scientist to do research, but the one that propelled Hugh Herr is exceedingly personal. For Herr, who is doing some of the world's most cutting-edge research on prostheses for amputees, it was the untimely death of a man he had never met.

In 1982, at the age of 17, Herr and a friend set out to climb Mount Washington in New Hampshire. They were caught in a snowstorm after losing their way in temperatures of -20°F (-28.8°C) and whiteout conditions. Against all odds, the two were finally rescued after three and a half days. Herr's legs were so damaged by the cold that eventually they had to be amputated.

He learned later that a volunteer member of the rescue team, 28-year-old Albert Dow, had been killed in an avalanche during the search. Sad and angry over the death of a man who had died trying to save him, Herr embarked on an effort to enrich the lives of amputees. It is his way of honoring Dow. "I feel a responsibility to use my intellect and resources to do as much as I can to help people," he says. "That's Albert Dow's legacy for me."

Quoted in Andy Greenberg, "A Step Beyond Human," *Forbes*, December 14, 2009. www.forbes.com.

Though the use of MSCs to repair spinal injuries may be far in the future, a great deal of evidence indicates that in the near future more and more athletes will be seeking this type of treatment, especially for knee and shoulder injuries. According to Lehman, the research that has been done has erased doubts about the procedure. "Early on, there was a concern [about using stem cells]. Truth of the matter is, we are far enough down the line, and we . . . don't see a lot of negatives. We've got enough under our belt now where we are confident in using them."[76]

An Answer to Spinal Cord Injuries?

Some researchers are tackling one of the most profound injuries that can occur to an athlete—a spinal cord injury, or SCI. In the United States, between 1,500 and 2,500 people each year sustain SCIs playing sports. Work being done at the Mayo Clinic in 2012 may someday allow those who are totally or partially paralyzed because of spinal injuries to walk or possibly even play sports again.

The work of Mayo Clinic's neurologist and molecular scientist Anthony Windebank and spine surgeon and chemical engineer Michael Yaszemski is based on the knowledge that spinal cord fibers do have the capacity to regenerate. What is unknown is how to go about orchestrating that regeneration. One solution might be the use of Schwann cells, which are cells that can promote nerve growth. Researchers have been trying to determine how to stimulate the Schwann cells, which are found outside of the brain and spinal cord, to move to the site of the spinal injury. They are also unsure about how to create the right environment for nerve regeneration along a badly damaged spinal cord.

In a recent experiment, scientists anesthetized a rat and removed a small section of its spine to simulate a spinal cord injury. Yaszemski created a special scaffold—a tiny ladder-shaped frame upon which the nerves can regenerate. The scaffold also provided a portal through which the sci-

> ### scaffold
>
> A tiny ladder-like frame placed in a damaged spinal cord on which new nerve cells may grow.

entists could inject Schwann cells (harvested from the rat's blood) and drugs to speed healing. Yaszemski's scaffold was biodegradable, so that as the nerves regenerated, the scaffold did not have to be surgically removed. Instead, it simply dissolved to make room for the growing spinal cord.

Three months after the experiment began, the research team was elated to see as many as 5,000 new nerve cells growing along the length of the scaffold. The study demonstrated that nerves can regenerate with the right scaffold placed in the spinal cord system. Researchers hope this will someday lead to the healing of athletes and others with severe spinal injuries.

Though the success is one step in a very long, complex process, Windebank and Yaszemski are enthusiastic about the results of their research and the progress they have made. Though many challenges lie ahead, they believe they are on the right track. "I am optimistic that we will be conducting human clinical trials within ten years," Windebank says, adding, "This project is so exciting that I can't wait to get into the lab."[77]

A Thought-Propelled Prosthetic Arm

Other exciting research has to do with prosthetic limbs and their implications for amputees who want to live an active life. Prosthetic arms and hands have been especially difficult for research engineers. The human arm and hand make many different movements, from intricate tasks such as buttoning a shirt or tying a shoe to larger movements such as throwing a ball or carrying a package. These actions are accomplished because of the number and variety of muscles and joints found in the arm and hand.

For generations, people with prosthetic arms have been able to make just a few types of motions. Even with modern prostheses, movement tends to be slow. As a result, many arm amputees say they use their prostheses only for limited activities and rarely for athletics.

Amanda Kitts, a Knoxville, Tennessee, woman whose left arm was amputated after an automobile accident in 2006, was frustrated by the slowness of her prosthesis. To move the arm, she had to move her back muscles a particular way to make the wrist rotate. To move her elbow up or down, she had to flex her triceps and biceps. "It was a lot of work," she says. "It wasn't useful to me at all."[78]

targeted muscle reinnervation

Using the nerves of an amputated arm to help communicate signals to a myoelectric arm.

In 2009 Kitts agreed to take part in a research study on a prosthetic arm that is controlled by communication between the brain, muscles, and nerves. The procedure that makes that possible is a surgery called targeted muscle reinnervation, or TMR. Scientists believe it is the key to the way prostheses will be engineered in the future to benefit athletes as well as other arm amputees.

Targeted Muscle Reinnervation

The idea was pioneered by Todd Kuiken, director of the Neural Engineering Center for Artificial Limbs at the Rehabilitation Institute of Chicago. The basis of the idea is that the nerves of an amputated arm still exist. However, they are usually bundled at the stump end of the arm after amputation.

In TMR the surgeon unbundles those nerves and connects them to a muscle elsewhere in the body, usually a chest muscle. The surgeon then

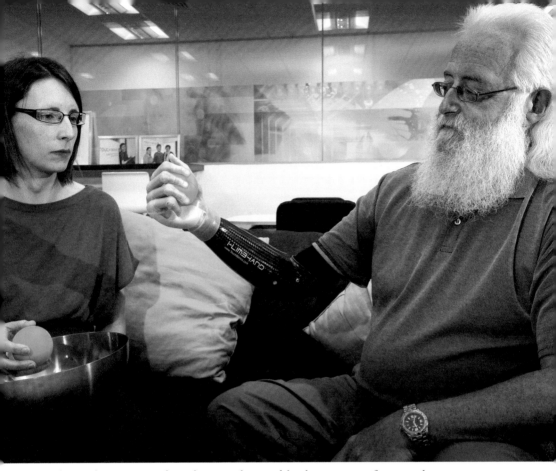

Electrodes connected to the muscles enable the wearer of a myoelectric prosthetic arm to move his wrist and open and close his hand around a ball. The prosthesis, which is one of the first with articulating fingers, represents a new generation of devices that might one day benefit athletes and others who have lost limbs.

places electrodes over that chest muscle. When a patient wants to move his or her arm, nerve signals are picked up by these electrodes and communicated to the myoelectric arm, telling it to move. In this way the chest muscles stimulate an electronic impulse to the patient's prosthetic arm.

As Katie Palmer of New York University's online magazine *Scienceline* explains, the nerves still have the capability of sending signals. "When a patient thinks about bending his elbow, the nerves to those muscles still fire, but instead of finding themselves at a dead end, they wind up in the chest, stimulating electrodes implanted above their pruned ends. The electrodes control the movement of the motorized prosthesis strapped to the patient's torso, and the artificial elbow bends."[79]

Research on TMR and its use with prostheses continues. Even though it is still a work in progress, Kitts says she has been delighted with the things she can do with her new prosthesis. She is delighted that she can play football with her son, change her baby's diapers, and accomplish dozens of other things she could not do with her prior prosthesis. "I'm able to move my hand, wrist, and elbow all at the same time," she says. "You think, and then your muscles move."[80]

Beyond Human?

Some of the most groundbreaking research in athletic prostheses is being led by Hugh Herr, director of the Biomechatronics Group at the MIT Media Lab. While many researchers are working to create more efficient and more lifelike prostheses for athletes, Herr is changing the idea that because an athlete uses a prosthesis it means that he or she is somehow handicapped. Herr, whose legs were both amputated when he was a teenager, envisions a future in which amputee athletes not only participate but dominate in their sports.

After the amputation of both of his legs, Herr threw himself into designing prostheses made especially for athletes. He decided early on that function was far more important than looks. He developed a variety of prostheses for various athletic activities—and some give him capabilities he never had with his own legs. Today, from his knees to the floor, he is all self-made. "I'm titanium, carbon, silicon, a bunch of nuts and bolts," he says. "My limbs that I wear have 5 computers, 12 sensors and muscle-like actuator systems that enable me to move throughout my day."[81]

Herr explains that as an athlete, he has a variety of prosthetic devices that he uses:

When you go into my closet, there are many, many pairs of legs. I have a running pair, I have a bionic walking pair, limbs that are waterproof. I have various legs to climb mountains and to descend steep ice walls, other feet that wedge into small rock fissures [and] others that stand on small rock edges the width of a coin. . . . My rock climbing feet are the size of baby feet. They're very, very small and very, very short so I can get the center of my body over my feet on a vertical wall.[82]

Spider Goats and Ligament Repair

For centuries scientists have marveled at the strength of spiderwebs—whose strands are more than five times stronger than steel and more elastic than nylon. That combination might make spiderweb silk a perfect material for creating artificial ligaments for athletes and others who have injured shoulders or knees.

The best spider-made silk, called dragline silk, is the particular strand spiders use to catch themselves as they fall. The problem is how to get large quantities of the spiderweb silk. Because spiders are cannibalistic they cannot be farmed.

Researchers have been working on a solution to this problem. In 2011 scientists at Utah State University successfully removed from a spider the gene that encodes dragline silk. They placed the gene into the DNA that prompts milk production in a goat's udder. This genetic information was then inserted into an egg and implanted into a mother goat named Freckles. When she lactates, her milk is full of spider-silk protein. The silk is then separated from the milk. The result is incredibly strong material that has already shown that it adapts well in the human body and does not cause inflammation or infection, as many other materials do. Scientists hope that in the near future they can begin creating and testing spider-made ligaments harvested from goat's milk.

Though many of Herr's inventions are years away from being available to the public, he believes that such innovative prostheses will eventually change the nature of sports. "If you're an amputee born today," he predicts, "there's a good chance that, in your 20s and 30s, your athletic performance will be augmented [beyond that of a nonamputee] and your daily life at least normalized."[83]

Herr foresees in the not-so-distant future that athletics for disabled people will draw bigger crowds than traditional sporting events, simply because of the advantages amputees will have over their sound-bodied peers. "They'll be so exciting that regular old arms and legs will seem dull," he says. "If the Paralympics accept advances in technology, there'll come a day when the Paralympics will be more popular than the Olympics. There'll be these insane human-machine events."[84]

For centuries, researchers have worked to find ways to keep athletes healthy and, in the case of injury, to help them heal and rehabilitate so that they can safely and quickly return to their sport. In the future, it may be that not only the athletes but the sports themselves will be affected and improved by the strides made by sports medicine researchers.

Source Notes

Introduction: Getting Back in the Game

1. Quoted in Jeremy Olson, "Coaches Assail Dangerous Youth Hockey Hits," *Minneapolis Star Tribune*, January 3, 2012. www.startribune.com.

2. Quoted in CBS Minnesota, "Minnesota Hockey Player, 16, Paralyzed During Game," January 2, 2012. http://minnesota.cbslocal.com.

3. Quoted in Michael Rose, "Surgeon: Jablonski 'Can't Expect Much Recovery,'" St.LouisParkPatch, January 5, 2012. http://stlouispark.patch.com.

4. Quoted in KARE 11, "Doctors Confirm Benilde–St. Margaret's Hockey Player Unable to Walk," January 5, 2012. www.kare11.com.

5. Quoted in US Department of Veterans Affairs, "VA Research Finds Possible Link Between Head Trauma and Chronic Traumatic Encephalopathy," press release. www.va.gov.

6. Quoted in Lisa Marshall, "Battle of Wounded Knees," *Colorado Business Magazine*, April 14, 2009. www.cobizmag.com.

7. Quoted in Marshall, "Battle of Wounded Knees."

Chapter One: What Is Sports Medicine?

8. Sam Alder, personal interview by author, December 22, 2011, Minneapolis, MN.

9. Alder, personal interview.

10. Alder, personal interview.

11. Quoted in D.W. Masterson, "The Ancient Greek Origins of Sports Medicine," *British Journal of Sports Medicine*, December 1976, p. 200.

12. Michael Grant, *Gladiators*. New York: Delacorte, 1967, pp. 49–50.

13. Greg Pfiefer, telephone interview by author, January 3, 2012.

14. Brady Harrison, personal interview by author, January 17, 2012, St. Paul, MN.

15. Harrison, personal interview.

16. Robert J. Henderson, "Microdiscectomy Surgery Video: A Spine Surgeon Explains the Procedure," video, Spine-Health. www.spine -health.com.

17. Quoted in Kelly Puente, "Wrestler, 17, Dies of Staph Infection," CafeMom, July 24, 2008. www.cafemom.com.

18. Jené Shaw, "Iron Docs," *Inside Triathlon*, March 9, 2012, p. 72.

19. Quoted in Shaw, "Iron Docs," p. 72.

Chapter Two: Concussion Research

20. Glenn Olsen, telephone interview by author, December 11, 2011.

21. Linda Carroll and David Rosner, *The Concussion Crisis: Anatomy of a Silent Epidemic.* New York: Simon and Schuster, 2011, pp. 10–11.

22. Eva Connor, personal interview by author, December 11, 2011.

23. Connor, personal interview.

24. Quoted in Jeffrey Kluger, "Headbanger Nation," *Time*, February 3, 2011. www.time.com.

25. Ken Adams, personal interview by author, February 21, 2012, St. Paul, MN.

26. Adams, personal interview.

27. Quoted in Christopher Nowinski, *Head Games*. Boston: Thought Leaders, 2011, p. 133.

28. Nowinski, *Head Games*, p. 132.

29. Quoted in Nowinski, *Head Games*, p. 72.

30. Carroll and Rosner, *The Concussion Crisis*, pp. 123–24.

31. Quoted in Steve Jansen and Gus Garcia-Roberts, "Knocked Out," *City Pages* (Minneapolis-St. Paul), August 17, 2011, p. 13.

32. Kluger, "Headbanger Nation."

33. Quoted in Ryan Jaslow, "Derek Boogaard Had Chronic Traumatic Encephalopathy When He Died: Report," healthpop, CBS News, December 6, 2011. www.cbsnews.com.

34. Quoted in Kluger, "Headbanger Nation."

Chapter Three: Overuse Injury

35. Donald Neally, telephone interview by author, February 1, 2012.

36. Frank Jobe, "Interview with Tommy John and Dr. Frank Jobe," radio podcast, Baseball Prospectus, June 14, 2009. www.baseballprospectus .com.

37. Jobe, "Interview with Tommy John and Dr. Frank Jobe."

38. Tommy John, "Interview with Tommy John and Dr. Frank Jobe," radio podcast, Baseball Prospectus, June 14, 2009. www.baseballpro spectus.com.

39. Tarek O. Souryal, telephone interview by author, February 3, 2012.

40. Quoted in ESPN Feature, "ACL Injury, ACL Tear, ACL Surgery," Texas Sports Medicine and Orthpaedic Group. www.txsportsmed .com.

41. Souryal, telephone interview.

42. Quoted in ESPN Feature, "ACL Injury, ACL Tear, ACL Surgery."

43. Quoted in ESPN Feature, "ACL Injury, ACL Tear, ACL Surgery."

44. Souryal, telephone interview.

45. Joseph Aiello, "History of Platelet-Rich Plasma Therapy," video, Health Videos. www.hivvids.com.

46. Quoted in David Epstein, "Sports Medicine's New Frontiers," *Sports Illustrated*, August 8, 2011, p. 48.

47. Quoted in Mayo Clinic, "Combo Treatment Helps Heal Overused, Aching Joints," January 17, 2012. www.mayoclinic.org.

48. Quoted in Alan Schwarz, "A Promising Treatment for Athletes, in Blood," *New York Times*, February 17, 2009. www.nytimes.com.

Chapter Four: Prosthetics Research

49. Quoted in LZ Granderson, "Scott Odom's Driven to Play Basketball," ESPN, October 14, 2011. http://espn.go.com.

50. Lily Lange, telephone interview by author, January 22, 2012.

51. Lange, telephone interview.

52. Eileen Malek, personal interview by author, February 9, 2012, River Falls, WI.

53. Anonymous, personal interview by author, February 3, 2012, Minneapolis, MN.

54. Anonymous, personal interview.

55. Becky Born, personal interview by author, February 10, 2012, Minneapolis, MN.

56. Born, personal interview.

57. Quoted in My Fox Houston, "Go, Go Gadget Putter! Scientists Testing Sport-Specific Limbs," www.myfoxhouston.com.

58. Quoted in My Fox Houston, "Go, Go Gadget Putter!"

59. Hector Picard, telephone interview by author, February 10, 2012.

60. Picard, telephone interview.

61. Quoted in Carol Pogash, "A Personal Call to a Prosthetic Invention," *New York Times*, July 2, 2008. www.nytimes.com.

62. Pogash, "A Personal Call to a Prosthetic Invention."

63. Quoted in Pogash, "A Personal Call to a Prosthetic Invention."

64. Quoted in Charles Kupperman, "Anticipating Amputation: The Case for Communication," *BioMechanics*, February 2003. http://ertlreconstruction.com.

65. Quoted in Alexander Wolff, "Prosthetics: Between Man and Machine," *Sports Illustrated*, August 8, 2011, p. 50.

66. Anonymous, personal interview.

67. Anonymous, personal interview.

Chapter Five: The Exciting Future of Sports Medicine

68. Michael K. Lee, personal interview by author, January 4, 2012, Minneapolis, MN.

69. Christophe Lenglet, personal interview by author, January 19, 2012, Minneapolis, MN.

70. Lenglet, personal interview.

71. Lenglet, personal interview.

72. Quoted in *Columbia Chronicle*, "The Future of Athletic Healing," September 6, 2011. http://columbiachronicle.com.

73. Quoted in *Columbia Chronicle*, "The Future of Athletic Healing."

74. Quoted in Bill Pennington, "Sports Medicine Turns to Stem Cell 'Repair Kits,'" *New York Times*, March 20, 2007. www.nytimes.com.

75. Quoted in Newswise, "Research Indicates That Adult Human Mesenchymal Stem Cells May Be Viable Treatment for Spinal Cord Injury Repair," October 5, 2011. www.newswise.com.

76. Quoted in *Columbia Chronicle*, "The Future of Athletic Healing."

77. Quoted in Mayo Clinic, "Spinal Cord Injury Research." http://discoverysedge.mayo.edu.

78. Quoted in Pam Belluck, "In New Procedure, Artificial Arm Listens to Brain," *New York Times*, February 10, 2009. www.nytimes.com.

79. Katie Palmer, "A Neuro-Engineer's Call to Arms: What Can the Next Generation of Artificial Limbs Teach Us About Our Bodies?," *Scienceline.* http://scienceline.org.

80. Quoted in Belluck, "In New Procedure, Artificial Arm Listens to Brain."

81. Quoted in NPR, "The Double Amputee Who Designs Better Limbs," *Fresh Air*, August 10, 2011. www.npr.org.

82. Quoted in NPR, "The Double Amputee Who Designs Better Limbs."

83. Quoted in Wolff, "Prosthetics: Between Man and Machine," p. 52.

84. Quoted in Wolff, "Prosthetics: Between Man and Machine," p. 53.

Facts About Sports Medicine Research

Prevalence of Sports Injuries

• According to the American Association of Neural Surgeons, 62,000 high school sports-related concussions occur each year in the United States.

• According to the Children's Hospital of Pittsburgh, 50 percent of children 14 and under treated for a bicycle injury are diagnosed with a brain injury.

• According to the American Association of Neural Surgeons, nearly 450,000 sports-related head injuries were treated in US emergency rooms in 2009.

• The Consumer Product Safety Commission says that 30,000 cheerleaders are treated at emergency rooms each year.

• According to the *Journal of Strength and Conditioning Research*, weight lifting is the sport with the fewest reported injuries, with .0013 injuries per 100 hours, while the most dangerous is rugby, with .8 injuries per 100 hours.

• Women college basketball players are six times more likely than men to suffer an ACL tear, according to the National Institute of Arthritis and Musculoskeletal and Skin Diseases.

• According to the National Institutes of Health, concussions make up 20 percent of all soccer injuries, and the actual number could be higher because so many concussions are unrecognized.

Repair and Prevention

• Some trainers in fifth-century BC Greece advocated an all-meat diet, sometimes recommending consumption of 20 pounds (9 kg) in one day, as a way of increasing an athlete's strength, says sports historian D.W. Masterson.

- According to the Arthritis Foundation, 650,000 arthroscopic surgeries are performed on knees in the United States each year.

- Chemists at the University of Bristol in England say that spider silk (a material that may be used to replace damaged human ligaments) is so strong that a pencil-width strand of the material would theoretically be enough to stop a Boeing 747 in flight.

- Todd Kuiken, who developed the process of targeted muscle reinnervation, reports a 96 percent success rate for the surgery.

- According to a 2010 report in Florida's *Gainesville Times*, the cost of having Tommy John surgery can be $15,000, not including the cost of rehabilitation afterward.

Rules, Laws, and Sports Medicine

- As of February 2012, 30 states plus the District of Columbia had enacted concussion legislation, informing athletes, parents, and coaches about concussions; removing an athlete from play or practice who seems to have suffered a concussion; and requiring clearance by a doctor before returning to play or practice.

- South African sprinter Oscar Pistorius, a double amputee, was banned from the 2008 Olympics because the IAAF (International Association of Athletics Federations) believed his Cheetah Flex-Foot prostheses would give him an unfair advantage over sound-bodied competitors.

- According to the NFL's Head, Neck and Spine Committee, the league's rule moving the kickoff line up 5 yards to the 35-yard line reduced concussions by 50 percent in 2011 due to the lack of a running start by kickoff returners.

- After the illegal check that caused the traumatic spinal injury to Jack Jablonski, Minnesota high school hockey officials increased the penalty for such a check from two minutes to five, and possibly a game suspension.

Spinal Cord Injuries

- The Spinal Injury Network says that two-thirds of those with spinal injuries who can feel a needlestick in their legs eventually will get enough leg strength to be able to walk again.

- According to the National Spinal Cord Injury Association, about 7,800 spinal cord injuries occur in the United States each year, with 12 percent of these injuries resulting from sports-related activities.

- Approximately 66 percent of sports-related spinal cord injuries are caused by diving, according to the National Spinal Cord Injury Association.

Related Organizations

American College of Sports Medicine (ACSM)
401 W. Michigan St.
Indianapolis, IN 46202-3233
phone: (317) 637-9200
website: www.acsm.org

The ACSM is made up of more than 20,000 doctors, trainers, physical therapists, and researchers who treat and study sports injuries. Visitors to the website will find many resources about sports injuries under the link "News and Publications." That link contains many updates about ongoing research and advances in sports medicine.

American Medical Society for Sports Medicine (AMSSM)
4000 W. 114th St., Suite 100
Leawood, KS 66211
phone: (913) 327-1415
website: www.amssm.org

This organization's purpose is to foster a close relationship among dedicated, competent sports medicine specialists, to provide a forum for sharing of information, and to encourage and support research in the area of sports medicine.

Brain Injury Association of America (BIAA)
1608 Spring Hill Rd., Suite 110
Vienna, VA 22182
phone: 800-444-6443
website: www.biausa.org

The BIAA is the largest and oldest brain injury organization in the United States. It offers education, research, and advocacy for people with brain injury, their families and friends, as well as health care professionals. Its National Directory of Brain Injury Services offers a comprehensive online directory of TBI (traumatic brain injury) health providers.

RELATED ORGANIZATIONS

CDC's National Center for Injury Prevention & Control
4770 Buford Hwy. NE
Mail Stop F-63
Atlanta, GA 30341
phone: (800) 232-4636
website: www.cdc.gov

The CDC website provides thorough and up-to-date information on concussions and other brain injuries, as well as links to downloads, including "Heads Up on Concussion" toolkits. It also offers free guides and other educational information about proper ways to recognize concussions.

National Athletic Trainers' Association (NATA)
2952 Stemmons Fwy.
Dallas, TX 75247
phone: (214) 637-6282
website: www.nata.org

This organization works closely with physical therapists and physicians to help athletes with rehabilitation after injuries. The NATA's website has an extensive glossary of sports injury terms that may be downloaded.

Society for Neuroscience
1121 Fourteenth St. NW, Suite 1010
Washington, DC 20005
phone: (202) 962-4000
website: www.sfn.org

The Society for Neuroscience is an organization of scientists and physicians throughout the world whose research is focused on the study of the brain and nervous system.

Spinal Cord Society (SCS)
19051 County Hwy. 1
Fergus Falls, MN 56537-7609
phone: (218) 739-5252
website: www.spinalcordsociety.com

This is a national organization founded in 1978 because of dissatisfaction with the direction of spinal cord treatment and research. Rather than emphasizing the care of those with spinal cord injuries, the SCS encourages and supports research dedicated to curing such injuries. The SCS publishes a monthly newsletter.

Sports Legacy Institute (SLI)
PO Box 181225
Boston, MA 02118
phone: (781) 262-3324
website: www.sportslegacy.org

The goal of the SLI is education and increased awareness in the athletic and medical communities about the dangers of concussions. Its website has videos detailing the causes of concussions, excellent photographs showing brains with tau protein tangles, and links to research sites and analysis of the latest concussion news and ongoing research.

For Further Research

Books

Linda Bickerstaff, *Frequently Asked Questions About Concussions*. New York: Rosen, 2010.

Peter Brukner and Karim Khan, *Clinical Sports Medicine*. Australia: McGraw-Hill, 2010.

Linda Carroll and David Rosner, *The Concussion Crisis: Anatomy of a Silent Epidemic*. New York: Simon and Schuster, 2011.

Lauri S. Friedman and Hal Marcovitz, *Is Stem Cell Research Necessary?* San Diego, CA: ReferencePoint, 2010.

Mary-Lane Kamberg, *Sports Concussions*. New York: Rosen, 2011.

Hal Marcovitz, *Stem Cell Research*. San Diego, CA: ReferencePoint, 2011.

Christopher Nowinski, *Head Games: Football's Concussion Crisis*. Boston: Thought Leaders, 2011.

Periodicals

Erik Brady, "Making an Impact in Concussion Research: UNC's Guskiewicz on Cutting Edge," *USA Today*, November 22, 2011.

Steve Jansen and Gus Garcia-Roberts, "Knocked Out," *City Pages* (Minneapolis-St. Paul), August 17, 2011.

Michael Sokolov, "The Fast Life of Oscar Pistorius," *New York Times*, January 18, 2012.

Websites

Amputee Coalition (www.amputee-coalition.org/research_participation .html). The Amputee Coalition develops educational resources, booklets, videos, and fact sheets to enhance the knowledge and coping skills of people affected by amputation. Its website has links to the latest prosthetic research, as well as research opportunities for amputees to become involved in future research studies.

Biomechatronics Group (http://biomech.media.mit.edu). The Biome-chatronics Group (BG), directed by Hugh Herr, is part of the Massachusetts Institute of Technology's Media Lab. Its website features articles about new designs for prostheses and other research that can benefit not only amputees but sound-bodied people, too. The site also has a link to an excellent video about the work BG does.

Medline Plus: Sports Injuries (www.lm.nih.gov/medlineplus/sport sinjuries.html). This website is maintained by National Institutes of Health's National Library of Medicine. It has extensive information on muscle sprains, ACL injuries, rotator cuff injuries, and many other sports injuries. It also provides links to articles explaining new research pertaining to athletic injuries.

oandp.com (www.oandp.com). This website is a resource for orthotics (devices to help straighten or control a body part) and prosthetics information. It has links to information about new prostheses for children, clinical studies about new procedures in sports medicine, as well as reports on upcoming research projects involving orthotics and prosthetics.

On Being a Scientist: A Guide to Responsible Conduct in Research (www.nap.edu/openbook.php?record_id=12192&page=R1). This free, downloadable book from the National Academy of Sciences Committee on Science, Engineering, and Public Policy provides a clear explanation of the responsible conduct of scientific research. The book offers invaluable insights for student researchers.

Index

Note: Boldface page numbers indicate illustrations.

INDEX

sports, growth in participation, 17

sports medicine history, 15–17

sports medicine specialties, 17

staph infections, 20–21, **21**

stem cells, 65–68

sub-concussive hits, 34, 35–36

surgery, 19, 20, 40–45, **43**

targeted muscle reinnervation (TMR), 70–72, **71**

tau proteins, 32

teenagers. *See* youth

tendons

  arthroscopy to repair, 43

  defined, 40

  PPR therapy to speed healing of, 48–49

  replacement of ligament with, 42

  transplants of, 40, 42

tennis injuries to knees, 42–44, 45–47

tenotomy, 48

terminal devices (TDs), 55

thought-propelled protheses, 70–72, **71**

Time (magazine), 35

Tommy John surgery, 42, 44, 66

traumatic brain injuries, 12

  See also concussions

treatments

  ancient, 15

  platelet-rich plasma injection, 47–49

rest, 38, 40

stem cell injection, 66

surgery, 19, 20, 40–45, **43**

tenotomy, 48

workout routine adjustments, 38, 41

See also protheses

triathlons, 22–23, 59

TRS, 55, 56

ulnar collateral ligament (UCL)

  cause of injuries to, 40

  described, 39

  sufferers of, 40

  surgery for, 40–42, 44

Verduyn, Pieter, 52

Ward, Hines, 48

Waters, Andre, 32

Webster, Martell, 19–20

Webster, Mike, 31

Windebank, Anthony, 69

woodpecker study, 33

Woods, Tiger, 48

workout routine adjustments, 38, 41

wrestling injuries, 18–19

X-rays, MRIs compared to, 19

Yaszemski, Michael, 69

youth

  ACL injuries, 46–47

Picture Credits

Cover: © iStockphoto.com

AP Images: 11, 16, 31, 35, 39, 53, 60, 64

Patrick Farrell/MCT/Landov: 57

Simon Fraser/Science Photo Library: 67

Dr. P. Marazzi/Science Photo Library: 21

Philippe Psaila/Science Photo Library: 71

Thinkstock/Comstock: 8

Thinkstock/Digital Vision: 9 (top)

Thinkstock/iStockphoto.com: 9 (bottom)

Jim Varney/Science Photo Library: 43

Steve Zmina: 27

PICTURE CREDITS

About the Author

Gail Stewart is the award-winning author of more than 250 books for teens and young adults. The mother of three grown sons, she and her husband live in Minneapolis, Minnesota.